T0130808

Current Concepts in Flatfoot Deformity

Editor

JARRETT D. CAIN

CLINICS IN PODIATRIC MEDICINE AND SURGERY

www.podiatric.theclinics.com

Consulting Editor
THOMAS J. CHANG

April 2023 • Volume 40 • Number 2

ELSEVIER

1600 John F. Kennedy Boulevard • Suite 1800 • Philadelphia, Pennsylvania, 19103-2899

http://www.theclinics.com

CLINICS IN PODIATRIC MEDICINE AND SURGERY Volume 40, Number 2
April 2023 ISSN 0891-8422, ISBN-13: 978-0-323-96179-0

Editor: Megan Ashdown
Developmental Editor: Arlene Campos

Clinics in Podiatric Medicine and Surgery (ISSN 0891-8422) is published quarterly by Elsevier Inc., 360 Park Avenue South, New York, NY 10010-1710. Months of issue are January, April, July, and October. Business and Editorial Offices: 1600 John F. Kennedy Blvd., Ste. 1800, Philadelphia, PA 19103-2899. Customer Service Office: 3251 Riverport Lane, Maryland Heights, MO 63043. Periodicals postage paid at New York, NY and additional mailing offices. Subscription prices are $329.00 per year for US individuals, $625.00 per year for US institutions, $100.00 per year for US students and residents, $405.00 per year for Canadian individuals, $754.00 for Canadian institutions, $490.00 for international individuals, $754.00 per year for international institutions, $100.00 per year for Canadian students/residents, and $220.00 per year for foreign students/residents. To receive student/resident rate, orders must be accompanied by name of affiliated institution, date of term, and the *signature* of program/residency coordinator on institution letterhead. Orders will be billed at individual rate until proof of status is received. Foreign air speed delivery is included in all *Clinics* subscription prices. All prices are subject to change without notice. POSTMASTER: Send address changes to *Clinics in Podiatric Medicine and Surgery*, Elsevier Health Sciences Division, Subscription Customer Service, 3251 Riverport Lane, Maryland Heights, MO 63043. **Customer Service: 1-800-654-2452 (US). From outside of the US, call 314-447-8871. Fax: 314-447-8029. E-mail: JournalsCustomerService-usa@elsevier.com (for print support); JournalsOnlineSupport-usa@elsevier.com (for online support).**

Reprints. For copies of 100 or more of articles in this publication, please contact the Commercial Reprints Department, Elsevier Inc., 360 Park Avenue South, New York, NY 10010-1710. Tel.: 212-633-3874; Fax: 212-633-3820; E-mail: reprints@elsevier.com.

Clinics in Podiatric Medicine and Surgery is covered in *MEDLINE/PubMed (Index Medicus)* and *EMBASE/Excerpta Medica.*

Contributors

CONSULTING EDITOR

THOMAS J. CHANG, DPM
Sonoma County Orthopedic/Podiatric Specialists, Santa Rosa, California

EDITOR

JARRETT D. CAIN, DPM, MSc
Associate Professor, Department of Orthopaedic Surgery, University of Pittsburgh School of Medicine, University of Pittsburgh Physicians, Comprehensive Foot and Ankle Center, Pittsburgh, Pennsylvania

AUTHORS

PATRICK R. BURNS, DPM
Assistant Professor of Orthopedic Surgery, University of Pittsburgh School of Medicine, University of Pittsburgh Physicians, Comprehensive Foot and Ankle Center, Pittsburgh, Pennsylvania

MARK J. CAPUZZI, DPM, AACFAS
Fellow, Current Fellow, Pennsylvania Intensive Lower Extremity Fellowship Program, Foot and Ankle Surgery, Premier Orthopedics/Pennsylvania Orthopaedic Center, Malvern, Pennsylvania

ALAN CATANZARITI, DPM, FACFAS
Program Director for West Penn Hospital Foot and Ankle Surgery, Section Chief for Podiatry, Department of Orthopedics, Allegheny Health Network, West Penn Hospital, Foot and Ankle Institute, Pittsburgh, Pennsylvania

MATTHEW COBB, DPM
Albuquerque, New Mexico

MATTHEW J. JOHNSON, DPM
Assistant Professor, Department of Orthopaedic Surgery, The University of Texas Southwestern Medical Center, Dallas, Texas

CRAIG E. KRCAL JR. DPM
Resident, Kaiser San Francisco Bay Area Foot and Ankle Residency Program, Oakland, California

KELLY KUGACH, DPM
Carilion Clinic, Institute for Orthopaedics and Neurosciences, Roanoke, Virginia

GEORGE TYE LIU, DPM
Assistant Professor, Department of Orthopaedic Surgery, The University of Texas Southwestern Medical Center, Dallas, Texas

SEAN R. LYONS, DPM
Resident PGY-3, Inova Fairfax Medical Campus, Fairfax, Virginia

CAITLIN MAHAN MADDEN, DPM, FACFAS
Private Practice, West Chester, Pennsylvania

KIERAN T. MAHAN, DPM, FACFAS, FCPP
Professor Emeritus, Department of Surgery, Temple University School of Podiatric Medicine

KSHITIJ MANCHANDA, MD
Assistant Professor, Department of Orthopaedic Surgery, The University of Texas Southwestern Medical Center, Dallas, Texas

JEFFREY M. MANWAY, DPM
Chief, Podiatry Section, UPMC Mercy Hospital, Program Director, UPMC Mercy Podiatric Surgical Residency, Clinical Instructor, University of Pittsburgh School of Medicine, Division of Foot and Ankle Surgery, UPP Department of Orthopedic Surgery, Monroeville, Pennsylvania

SARA MATEEN, DPM, AACFAS
Fellow, Foot and Ankle Deformity and Orthoplastics, Rubin Institute for Advanced Orthopedics, Baltimore, Maryland

ANDREW J. MEYR, DPM, FACFAS
Clinical Professor, Department of Podiatric Surgery, Temple University School of Podiatric Medicine, Philadelphia, Pennsylvania

JASON R. MILLER, DPM
Director, Pennsylvania Intensive Lower Extremity Fellowship Program, Foot and Ankle Surgery, Premier Orthopedics/Pennsylvania Orthopaedic Center, Malvern, Pennsylvania; Surgical Residency Program, Adjunct Associate Professor, Department of Surgery, Residency Director, Tower Health/Phoenixville Hospital Podiatric Medicine, PMSR/RRA, Temple University, Phoenixville, Pennsylvania

JASON V. NALDO, DPM, FACFAS
Assistant Professor, Department of Orthopaedics, Virginia Tech Carilion, School of Medicine, Carilion Clinic Institute for Orthopaedics and Neurosciences, Christiansburg, Virginia

SANDEEP PATEL, DPM
Chief of Podiatric Surgery, Diablo Service Area, Kaiser Permanente, Walnut Creek, California; Attending Staff, Kaiser San Francisco Bay Area, Foot and Ankle Residency Program, Oakland, California

NICHOLAS S. POWERS, DPM
Assistant Professor, Department of Orthopaedic Surgery, Atrium Health Wake Forest Baptist, Wake Forest University School of Medicine, Winston-Salem, North Carolina

ROLAND RAMDASS, DPM, FACFAS
Foot and Ankle Center, P.C., Winchester, Virginia; Residency Training Committee Inova Fairfax Medical Campus

KATHERINE M. RASPOVIC, DPM
Assistant Professor, Department of Orthopaedic Surgery, The University of Texas Southwestern Medical Center, Dallas, Texas

MADISON RAVINE, DPM
Clinical Fellow in Surgery, Cambridge Health Alliance, Harvard Medical School, Cambridge, Massachusetts

SCOTT SCHLEUNES, DPM
Resident Physician, Department of Orthopedics, Division of Foot and Ankle Surgery, West Penn Hospital, Pittsburgh, Pennsylvania

JOHN M. SCHUBERTH, DPM
Kaiser San Francisco Bay Area, Foot and Ankle Residency Program, Oakland, California; Department of Orthopedic Surgery, San Francisco, California

TYMOTEUSZ SIWY, DPM
Surgical Residency Program, PGY-2, Resident, Tower Health/Phoenixville Hospital Podiatric Medicine and Surgery Residency, PMSR/RRA, Phoenixville, Pennsylvania

DEVRIE STELLAR, DPM
Resident PGY-3, Inova Fairfax Medical Campus, Fairfax, Virginia

MICHAEL H. THEODOULOU, DPM, FACFAS
Chief, Division of Podiatric Surgery, Cambridge Health Alliance, Harvard Medical School, Cambridge, Massachusetts

JENNIFER C. VAN, DPM, MBA, FACFAS, FACPM
Chair and Clinical Assistant Professor, Department of Podiatric Surgery, Temple University School of Podiatric Medicine, Philadelphia, Pennsylvania

MICHAEL D. VAN PELT, DPM
Assistant Professor, Department of Orthopaedic Surgery, The University of Texas Southwestern Medical Center, Dallas, Texas

DANE K. WUKICH, MD
Professor and Chair, Department of Orthopaedic Surgery, The University of Texas Southwestern Medical Center, Dallas, Texas

Contents

Anatomic and Biomechanical Considerations of Flatfoot Deformity   239

Michael H. Theodoulou and Madison Ravine

> In this article, the authors present essential anatomy in the presence of the postural flat foot. There is a recognition of static versus dynamic stabilizers of the foot. In the continuum of the collapsed foot, there is an exploration of anatomic and pathologic changes. Providing this fundamental knowledge will allow the reader to appreciate the disease process to establish a prognosis and consider treatment alternatives.

The Role of Equinus in Flatfoot Deformity   247

Devrie Stellar, Sean R. Lyons, Roland Ramdass, and Andrew J. Meyr

> Equinus plays an important role in flatfoot deformity. Proper evaluation and surgical management are critical to comprehensively treat and successfully resolved patients' symptoms. We have discussed the cause, evaluation, and some of the common surgical options. Each procedure has its inherent benefits and risks. It is imperative that the foot and ankle surgeon identify and include these procedures as part of the complete reconstructive surgery.

Single and Double Osteotomies of the Calcaneus for the Treatment of Posterior Tibial Tendon Dysfunction   261

Jeffrey M. Manway

> Posterior tibial tendon disfunction is one of the most commonly treated foot and ankle entities. Surgical treatment may consist of various components and is often performed on an a-la-carte basis. Commonly, joint preservative surgery for posterior tibial tendon dysfunction invariably involves one or more osteotomies of the calcaneus. This article evaluates the current existing evidence guiding providers in the selection of single or double calcaneal osteotomies.

Addressing Medial Column Instability in Flatfoot Deformity   271

Scott Schleunes and Alan Catanzariti

> A stable medial column is important to the normal function of the foot and ankle. Medial column instability and forefoot varus can result in compensatory hindfoot motion leading to stress along the medial soft-tissue

structures. Medial column stabilization should therefore be considered when (1) forefoot varus deformity is identified following hindfoot realignment; (2) pronounced medial column instability is present, even in the absence of forefoot varus; and (3) when degenerative changes are present within the medial column articulations. Common surgical procedures include arthrodesis of the talonavicular joint, naviculocuneiform joint, and first tarsometatarsal joint, as well as osteotomy of the medial cuneiform (Cotton osteotomy).

The adult-acquired flatfoot is a complex multiplanar deformity that requires the foot and ankle surgeon to balance soft tissue, correct hindfoot valgus, and address instability of the medial column. The naviculocuneiform joint is historically underappreciated in regard to its involvement in medial column instability relative to the talonavicular and tarsometatarsal joints. Proper clinical and radiographic evaluation of the medial column, specifically evaluating for deformity at each medial column joint, will allow the surgeon to ensure correction of deformity and decrease the recurrence of instability or failure of the reconstruction.

The objective of this article was to review the deltoid ligament and spring ligament specifically as they pertain to ligament insufficiency and adult-acquired flatfoot deformity. Discussion includes the normal and abnormal biomechanical forces that extend through these ligaments in normal and flatfoot deformity. Current literature related to spring ligament repair as part of the flatfoot deformity reconstruction is also reviewed.

Different types of arthrodesis for flatfoot deformity have a long history in foot and ankle surgery. Arthrodesis of the rearfoot can be a useful tool in helping correct deformity and maintaining that correction with good long-term results. Questions have risen recently however about the necessity of including the calcaneocuboid joint in the traditional rearfoot arthrodesis or triple arthrodesis. The double arthrodesis of the talonavicular and subtalar joints has grown in popularity and this review helps the reader choose with a review of the biomechanics, surgical approaches, fixation techniques and recent literature outcomes of both procedures.

Rigid flatfoot deformity with valgus ankle instability is a complex condition to treat. Thorough clinical and radiographic evaluation is vital to determine treatment strategies. Nonoperative treatment usually relies on bracing or various orthoses. Surgical interventions include ligament reconstruction, osteotomies, arthrodesis, arthroplasty, or a combination of these procedures. Before addressing the ankle deformity, a plantigrade foot is important so a staged approach may be necessary. Misalignment of the ankle replacement can lead to edge loading and early failure. As the implants and our understanding of ankle arthroplasty improve, more patients may benefit from a motion-preserving procedure rather than an arthrodesis.

Adult acquired flatfoot is a progressive deformity of the foot and ankle, which frequently becomes increasingly symptomatic. The posterior tibial tendon is most commonly associated with the deformity. A targeted physical examination with plain film radiographs is the recommended initial assessment, which will further guide a physician toward procuring more advanced imaging or toward surgical intervention. In this chapter the authors review the current literature of their approach to the treatment of the ankle in end stage of adult acquired flatfoot deformity.

Reconstructive surgery of the symptomatic pes planus deformity is a very common procedure with relatively good outcomes. Many factors such as patient selection, patient expectations, and surgical execution can influence the results. In addition to achieving osseous union, the overall postoperative alignment is critical in determining functional outcome. Specifically, under- and over-correction respectively present their own unique problems and symptomatology. The purpose of this review is to discuss the adverse outcomes after mal-reduction of flatfoot reconstruction and emphasize the strategies to correct the subsequent deformity.

The pediatric flatfoot can include multiple planes of deformity and concomitant concerns such as metatarsus adductus and equinus. Each aspect of the deformity must be carefully evaluated before any surgical planning. The goal of surgery should be an improvement in symptoms by creating a controllable foot with a reduction of deforming forces. There are multiple procedures that can be used for the pediatric flatfoot, including the Evans calcaneal osteotomy, the Cotton medial cuneiform osteotomy, the medial calcaneal slide osteotomy, and arthroereisis implants. Each contributes in a specific way to the overall deformity correction. Multiple options exist for grafts and hardware.

CLINICS IN PODIATRIC MEDICINE AND SURGERY

SERIES OF RELATED INTEREST

Orthopedic Clinics
https://www.orthopedic.theclinics.com/
Clinics in Sports Medicine
https://www.sportsmed.theclinics.com/
Foot and Ankle Clinics
https://www.foot.theclinics.com/
Physical Medicine and Rehabilitation Clinics
https://www.pmr.theclinics.com/

THE CLINICS ARE AVAILABLE ONLINE!
Access your subscription at:
www.theclinics.com

Erratum: Author's name correction

In the published January 2023 issue of *Clinics in Podiatric Medicine and Surgery*, "Current Concepts in Sports Medicine" *Edited by Dr. Lawrence M. Oloff (Volume 40, Number 1),* one of the author's names was misspelled.

The author's name should be Ryan M. Sherick, not "Sherrick".

Clin Podiatr Med Surg 40 (2023) xi
https://doi.org/10.1016/j.cpm.2023.01.002
0891-8422/23/© 2023 Elsevier Inc. All rights reserved.

podiatric.theclinics.com

Foreword

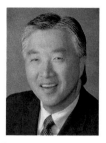

Thomas J. Chang, DPM
Consulting Editor

Ah…the topic of Flatfoot Surgery, and the debates never end. Nothing has garnered as much interest and discussion in the Foot and Ankle space over the past 20 years. Every scientific meeting on foot and ankle surgery includes a track on this topic. The study of the Flatfoot Deformity has spilled over into several other specialties, where researchers from basic science and biomechanics have published papers to further support or dispute our clinical outcomes.

As a young extern and resident in the late 1980s to the mid-1990s, I remember the majority of Flatfoot cases being managed with a triple arthrodesis. It was definitive and the standard at the time, yet came at a cost to movement. In a short time, there seemed to be a paradigm shift where the new question was "How could we get the same control of a triple arthrodesis by doing less?" The concept of double and single fusions started to be debated. As the distinction started between flexible and rigid deformities, the evolution of extra-articular osteotomies and joint salvage procedures became more popular. Soon thereafter, multiple joint-sparing procedures were used in combination versus fusions, and this debate continues today. Other common debates involve treating the medial versus the lateral column, soft tissue versus osseous procedures, isolated versus combination procedures, and the role of equinus, to name a few. The list goes on.

As our foot and ankle community has evolved in understanding the complexities of this deformity, our terminology and classification of Flatfoot have also matured. The literature has also reflected this evolution. In the 1970s, the commonplace term seemed to be Flatfoot Deformity. In the 1980s, the term Posterior Tibialis Tendon Dysfunction became more mainstream. Moving into the 1990s, the term Adult Acquired Flatfoot Deformity fell into favor. Shortly after, the Collapsing Pes Valgo Planus foot was often seen in describing this entity. Within the past few years, we have once again witnessed a change, the Progressive Collapsing Foot Deformity (PCFD). The recent Consensus statement on PCFD is another valuable addition to the conversation.

I felt it was time again for some continued discussion. Dr Cain has always shown passion for this topic. He has brought together a talented and richly experienced group

Clin Podiatr Med Surg 40 (2023) xiii–xiv
https://doi.org/10.1016/j.cpm.2023.01.001
0891-8422/23/© 2023 Published by Elsevier Inc.

podiatric.theclinics.com

of writers and created a valuable update to this timeless topic. I look forward to continuing the dialogue. I hope you enjoy this issue.

Thomas J. Chang, DPM
Sonoma County Orthopedic/
Podiatric Specialists
3536 Mendocino Avenue, Suite 300B
Santa Rosa, CA 95403, USA

E-mail address:
thomaschang14@comcast.net

Preface

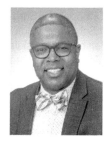

Jarrett D. Cain, DPM, MSc
Editor

Dr. Frederic Wood Jones affirmed from his work as an anatomist that *"every detail of the structure and function of the parts of the foot must be studied and realised for its own sake"*.[1] He stressed the significance and value of anatomic structures and function of the foot. This attention to detail is especially appreciated when it comes to evaluation of the flatfoot deformity.

Since the early work of Goldner et al,[2] Mann and Specht,[3] and Banks and McGlamry,[4] our understanding has evolved with classifications that have provided a framework for diagnosis and treatment of the condition. As our attention to anatomic structures has progressed, we continue to gain greater clarity in the diagnosis and treatment of flatfoot deformity.

To that end, the authors of this issue have contributed to further progress the scientific knowledge of flatfoot deformity. I extend heartfelt gratitude and appreciation for the

Clin Podiatr Med Surg 40 (2023) xv–xvi
https://doi.org/10.1016/j.cpm.2022.11.012
0891-8422/23/© 2022 Published by Elsevier Inc.

podiatric.theclinics.com

time, commitment, and expertise they so graciously shared in current concepts of flat-foot deformity in adults and children.

Jarrett D. Cain, DPM, MSc
Department of Orthopaedic Surgery
University of Pittsburgh School of Medicine
University of Pittsburgh Physicians
Comprehensive Foot & Ankle Center
1515 Locust Street #350
Pittsburgh, PA 15219, USA

E-mail address:
cain1074@gmail.com

REFERENCES

1. Wood Jones F. Structure and function as seen in the foot. London: Balliere, Tindall, and Cox; 1949. p. 1–4.
2. Goldner JL, Keats PK, Bassett FH 3rd, et al. Progressive talipes equinovalgus due to trauma or degeneration of the posterior tibial tendon and medial plantar ligaments. Orthop Clin North Am 1974;5(1):39–51. PMID: 4809543.
3. Mann RA, Specht LH. Posterior tibial tendon ruptures: analysis of eight cases. Foot Ankle 1982;2:350.
4. Banks AS, McGlamry ED. Tibialis posterior tendon rupture. J Am Podiatr Med Assoc 1987;77(4):170–6.

Anatomic and Biomechanical Considerations of Flatfoot Deformity

Michael H. Theodoulou, DPM, Madison Ravine, DPM*

KEYWORDS

- Pes planus • Flat foot • Collapsed foot • Posterior tibial tendon dysfunction
- Spring ligament • Equinus

KEY POINTS

- Anatomy of pediatric/adolescent versus adult.
- Static versus dynamic anatomy.
- Anatomy in the progression of the disease.
- Pathomechanics related to anatomic change.

INTRODUCTION

Pes planus, also known as pes planovalgus or colloquially termed flat foot or fallen arches, comprises a spectrum of deformities with many possible causes. This postural presentation may be developmental, such as a congenital pediatric flat foot, or acquired, as is the adult case acquired flat foot deformity. In simplistic terms, the flat foot deformity describes the common end-point of any abnormality that causes the medial longitudinal arch to collapse.[1] In its continuum, individuals may have symptomatic deformity from congenital pes planus deformity, which was previously asymptomatic. However, symptoms may progress to an adult acquired pes planus deformity, which results in the failure of various ligaments and tendons. As the degree of deformity progresses along a spectrum so does the clinical significance. This deformity may be relatively asymptomatic or lead to profound symptoms and dysfunction. Although some patients may compensate adequately to address the symptoms, others develop symptoms that are functionally debilitating. The most common subset of this deformity is adult acquired flat foot due to posterior tibial tendon dysfunction. The following article aims to provide a comprehensive review of flatfoot deformity, with a focus on

Cambridge Health Alliance, Harvard Medical School, 1493 Cambride Street, Cambridge, MA 02139, USA
* Corresponding author.
E-mail address: drtheodoulou@gmail.com

Clin Podiatr Med Surg 40 (2023) 239–246
https://doi.org/10.1016/j.cpm.2022.11.001
0891-8422/23/© 2022 Elsevier Inc. All rights reserved.

up-to-date anatomic and biomechanical considerations involved in the management of this deformity.

A REVIEW OF FUNCTIONAL ANATOMY

Three identified arches contribute to the inherent stability of the foot: the medial longitudinal arch, lateral longitudinal arch, and transverse arch. The medial longitudinal arch is composed of the bones and joints of the medial column, connected by strong plantar ligaments, namely the plantar calcaneonavicular or spring ligament.[1] The lateral longitudinal arch is composed of the lateral column, whereas the transverse arch runs transversely across the foot at the tarsometatarsal region of the foot.[2] Although in a flat foot deformity, the medial longitudinal arch is generally unstable, leading to flattening or collapse, it is essential to understand that all 3 arches of the foot are interconnected. The failure at 1 arch will inevitably lead to structural compromise at the other arches. Although the skeletal pedal architecture contributes to the overall stability of the foot, the extrinsic and intrinsic muscular and ligamentous structures are critical to maintaining this arch. We can further separate these components into static versus dynamic stabilizers, as discussed below and summarized in **Table 1**.

Dynamic Stabilizers

One of the most critical dynamic stabilizers of the hindfoot and medial column is the tibialis posterior tendon. Originating from the proximal tibia, fibula, and interosseous membrane, the tendon forms within the deep posterior compartment and passes posterior to the medial malleolus. It then trifurcates into its primary insertion along the navicular tuberosity and medial cuneiform. It also broadly and extensively inserts along the plantar aspect of the foot, across metatarsals 2 through 4, all 3 cuneiforms, the sustentaculum tali, and the cuboid, which further contributes to the extensive ligamentous support of the arch.[3,4] This tendon passes medial to the subtalar joint axis, thereby functioning as a supinatory force: inverting the subtalar joint, stabilizing the medial longitudinal arch, and plantarflexing the ankle joint. It serves throughout the gait cycle, decelerating subtalar joint pronation, preventing excess hindfoot eversion at heel contact, accelerating subtalar joint supination at midstance, and locking the midtarsal joint.[5] It also decelerates the lower leg's internal rotation.[3]

There are other extrinsic musculatures that provide dynamic support to the arch. Flexor digitorum longus also passes on the supinatory side of the subtalar joint axis. It spans the entire length of the plantar foot, inserting on the distal phalanges of the lesser digits. As the leg rotates during gait, tension generates on this tendon, which

Table 1	
Anatomic summary, stratified by dynamic versus static stabilizers as they function across the medial longitudinal arch	
Stabilization Class	**Structure**
Dynamic	Tibialis posterior
	Flexor digitorum longus
	Peroneus longus
	Tibialis anterior
	Peroneus brevis
Static	Spring ligament
	Deltoid ligament
Dynamic and Static	Plantar fascia
	Plantar intrinsics

contracts and supports the arch.[3] Furthermore, peroneus longus works to support the arch via plantarflexion of the first ray. As the tendon courses around the lateral malleolus, this creates a pulley mechanism through midstance into heel off, stabilizing the arch.

An assessment of functional anatomy would not be complete without mention of the appropriate muscular antagonists. The tibialis anterior, the antagonist to the peroneus longus, works to dorsiflex the first ray and also has a supinatory moment about the subtalar joint axis.[3] Peroneus brevis, the antagonist to the tibialis posterior, everts the subtalar joint and has a pronatory moment about the subtalar joint axis.[3]

Static Stabilizers

Although the extrinsic musculature provides necessary dynamic stabilization of the arch, there are static soft tissue stabilizers that work in concert to reinforce and maintain this arch. Because the posterior tibial tendon is the principal dynamic stabilizer, the spring ligament (or plantar calcaneonavicular ligament) is the primary static stabilizer of the medial longitudinal arch.[2,3,5] This ligament consists of the superomedial, medioplantar oblique, and inferoplantar longitudinal bundles (listed from medial to lateral). The superomedial bundle is the largest and most important of the three. It originates from the sustentaculum tali, passing below the talus, and finally inserts into the distal medial aspect of the navicular. This structure forms hammock-like support for the talar head, supporting the talonavicular joint.[2]

Forming a soft tissue confluence with the spring ligament and posterior tibial tendon is the deltoid ligament. This confluence works to prevent excessive talar head descent.[2] The deltoid ligament is further separated into deep and superficial components. The deep deltoid ligament stabilizes the tibiotalar articulation, resisting ankle valgus. The superficial deltoid ligament spans the subtalar and tibionavicular joints, limiting hindfoot eversion and medial talar head displacement.[2]

Other specific structures act as both dynamic and static stabilizers. The plantar fascia is considered both a static and dynamic stabilizer of the longitudinal arch. It originates from the tuberosity of the calcaneus and is composed of medial, central, and lateral bands spanning the entire length of the foot and inserting into the proximal phalanges. In a static sense, it prevents elongation of the plantar foot—much like a tie rod holding the anterior strut (lesser tarsus and metatarsals) and posterior strut (talus and calcaneus) together. As a dynamic stabilizer, it functions in the Windlass mechanism during the end of late stance. As the digits dorsiflex and the heel begins to leave the ground, the plantar fascia tenses, drawing the calcaneus and metatarsal heads toward one another to maintain the height of the medial longitudinal arch.[2,4] Although the plantar intrinsic musculature's role in stabilization is ill-defined, Basmajian and Stecko demonstrated through electromyographic studies that the intrinsic musculature is increasingly active in the static phase of gait in a pes planus foot as compared with a rectus foot.[3,6] Further hypotheses include that the intrinsics may work to sense deformation and provide local stabilization.[2] Other authors have hypothesized that the inherent orientation of the musculature, parallel to the long axis of the foot, provides support to the arch with contraction throughout gait.[3,5]

DEVELOPMENTAL CONSIDERATIONS

It is important to recall that flatfoot deformity may be congenital or acquired. Although there exists a period of skeletal development in which a certain degree of flatfoot is a normal finding. This postural presentation usually spontaneously resolves by ages 3 to 6 years, with the development of the pedal arches.[2] When this persists past the above-defined developmental period, it may be more characteristic of a congenital flatfoot deformity. In the congential deformity, specific malformations such as congenital cal-caneovalgus or congenital convex pes valgus, also known as vertical talus, may result in flexible and rigid flatfoot deformities.

There are many potential causes for pediatric flatfoot deformity whether congenital or acquired. This deformity may result from collagen disorders leading to ligamentous laxity, muscle-tendon imbalances, central and peripheral nerve pathologic condition, or even trauma. These may be due to congenital deformities, including the tarsal coa-lition, although this is typically asymptomatic until later in childhood or adolescence.[7,8] From a structural perspective, this may result from faulty biomechanical alignment of the lower extremity as the principal cause for a compensatory deformity of the foot. Suprapedal reasons include femoral anteversion, internal genicular position, internal tibial torsion, or equinus. Intrapedal causes for this may consist of forefoot varus lead-ing to compensatory pronation of the subtalar joint, flexible forefoot valgus, or meta-tarsus adductus to name a few.[3,7]

It is difficult to predict which of these pediatric flatfeet will progress to the symptom-atic pes planovalgus condition in the adult.[3] Literature reports that only approximately 7% to 15% of those with developmental flatfoot will eventually develop symptoms as adults that lead them to seek medical attention.[2,9] Regardless, a thorough under-standing of the developmental flatfoot is essential to distinguish the pathophysiology from the adult acquired flatfoot.

DETAILED DEVELOPMENT OF PATHOPHYSIOLOGY

The adult acquired flat foot deformity is the most common subset of pes planus defor-mity, with a reported incidence of greater than 3% in women aged older than 40 years and greater than 10% in all adults aged older than 65 years.[8,10,11] As previously mentioned, the posterior tibial tendon is the principal stabilizer of the medial longitu-dinal arch. Therefore, tendinopathy or dysfunction of this tendon is the most common cause of adult-acquired flatfoot. There is recognition of 4 stages of adult-acquired flat-foot. The classification was initially described in the 1980s by Johnson and Strom, later modified by Myerson to include Stage 4, and Stage 2 was further subdivided by Deland and colleagues.[10,12–16]

Stage 1

Stage 1 is characterized by posterior tibial tendon tenosynovitis or tendinosis in its mildest form, rather than frank degeneration of the tendon. The posterior tibial tendon is still intact with maintained motor function, able to invert the heel with the heel raise test. In this stage, pain or tenderness presents throughout the tendon; however, at this point, the length of the tendon is normal, and there may be minimal degeneration pre-sent. There may be mild weakness and minimal, flexible deformity appreciated as well. As such, treatment is generally conservative.[15]

Stage 2

As the pathologic condition advances, dysfunction and degeneration of the posterior tibial tendon progress, thereby leading to evident deformity and functional abnormal-ities. The posterior tibial tendon may be elongated or torn, and patients may or may not be able to perform a heel raise test on the affected side. Because the posterior tibial tendon degenerates and attenuates, its ability to actively invert the subtalar joint is weakened, compromising the ability to lock the midtarsal joint. Peroneus brevis, the muscular antagonist to the tibialis posterior, gains a mechanical advantage over the compromised posterior tibial tendon. This antagonism leads to eversion of the subtalar joint, midfoot pronation, and forefoot abduction at the transverse tarsal joint. The medial longitudinal arch further collapses as the heel begins to assume a valgus position and the forefoot abducts at the talonavicular joint.[15] There is a varying degree of forefoot supination resulting from an accommodation of the foot, permitting the medial and lateral column to remain in contact with the ground. At the same time, the hindfoot is in a valgus position. This medial instability will lead to sinus tarsi pain associated with subtalar impingement as the disease progresses.[14,15] With the talus now unsupported and plantarflexed and the dynamic stabilizers compromised, the spring ligament then undergoes a secondary attenuation. Furthermore, once the heel becomes lateralized and assumes a more valgus position, the pull of the triceps surae complex is also lateralized and begins to evert the calcaneus because it develops a pronatory moment across the subtalar joint axis.[15] This increased pronation is accentuated in underlying equinus deformity as well. It is essential to note the deformation remains supple and manually reducible on the physical examination at this point; however, standard weight-bearing radiographs will demonstrate a structural deformity.

In 2006, Deland and colleagues subdivided stage 2 into stage 2A and stage 2B. Stage 2A was described as increased heel valgus but minimal abduction through the midfoot as determined by clinical and radiographic examination. In contrast, stage 2B was described as increased heel valgus with greater than 30% uncovering of the talonavicular head as seen on weight-bearing anteroposterior radiographs of the foot.[16] Deland and colleagues noted that due to this distinction, stage 2A might benefit from the medial calcaneal slide procedure, whereas stage 2B may benefit from lateral column lengthening as well.[16] Operative treatment in this stage generally depends on the severity of the deformity seen. Commonly joint-sparing procedures are used. Depending on the amount of pathologic condition to the posterior tibial tendon, an adjunct tendon transfer may be performed, most commonly, transfer of the flexor digitorum longus tendon to the navicular tuberosity. Further, depending on the degree of forefoot supinatus, a medial cuneiform opening wedge may be used.[14]

Stage 3

A Stage 3 deformity signifies a more rigid deformity, which generally develops as a function of time. At this point, the deformation is no longer flexible and manually reducible. There is commonly complete disruption of the posterior tibial tendon. The static stabilizers, namely the spring ligament, are attenuated or even disrupted at this point. The hindfoot is in a fixed valgus position, with the forefoot abducted. Pain is generally due to degenerative changes at the triple joint complex (talonavicular, calcaneocuboid, subtalar joint). Patients may begin to develop secondary pain laterally, near the sinus tarsi or subfibular region due to impingement because the foot is rigidly valgus. In this presentation, joint destructive procedures, including double or triple arthrodesis, are frequently used. A Stage 3 deformity is demonstrated in **Fig. 1**.

Stage 4

The final most severe stage of deformity is characterized by valgus angulation and talar tilt of the ankle joint with associated deltoid ligament insufficiency. This malalignment may lead to early degeneration of the ankle joint.[15] In nonpathological functional anatomy, the deltoid ligament provides significant stabilization to the medial aspect of the tibiotalocalcaneal joint complex; however, because the deformity progresses, this becomes attenuated valgus malalignment. Damage to the deltoid ligament is usually limited to the superficial component. However, damage to the deep ligaments can be

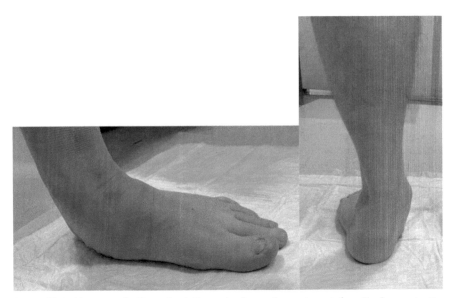

Fig. 1. Clinical images of a Stage 3 adult acquired pes planovalgus deformity demonstrating hindfoot valgus and complete collapse of the medial longitudinal arch.

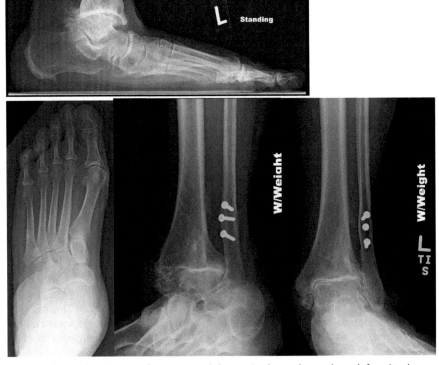

Fig. 2. Radiographic images of a Stage 4 adult acquired pes planovalgus deformity demonstrating ankle valgus and degenerative changes at the ankle joint.

seen in the late process.[2] This stage is further subdivided into a flexible ankle deformity with minimal arthritic changes versus advanced, rigid, and degenerative. A severe Stage 4 deformity is seen in **Fig. 2**. The early deformity may be amenable to deltoid ligament reconstruction with a triple arthrodesis. However, treatment is complex in a fixed ankle valgus deformity and may be limited to a tibiotalocalcaneal fusion versus total ankle arthroplasty with an implant.[14]

CLINICAL CARE POINTS

- The anatomy of the pediatric and adult flatfoot deformity are important in understanding its biomechanics and pathology of deformity.
- As the pathology progresses, it is important to distinguish between the static and dynamic contributors of the flatfoot deformity.
- As the flatfoot deformity, it is important to understand the anatomic changes as it relates to the pathomechanics.

SUMMARY

The appreciation of pathoanatomy as it presents in pediatric/adolescent and acquired collapsed foot remains crucial in understanding the disease process and its progression through secondary pathomechanics. The reader can enjoy a more significant experience of used diagnostic and treatment measures in its management with this understanding.

REFERENCES

1. Van Boerum DH, Sangeorzan BJ. Biomechanics and pathophysiology of flat foot. Foot Ankle Clin N Am 2003;8:419–30.
2. Flores DV, Gomez CM, Davis MA, et al. Adult acquired flatfoot deformity: anatomy, biomechanics, staging, and imaging findings. Radiographics 2019;39(5):1437–60.
3. Mahan KT, Flanigan KP. Chapter 44: flexible valgus deformity. McGlamry's comprehensive textbook of foot and ankle surgery. 4th edition. Philadelphia: Lippincott Williams & Wilkins; 2012. p. 585–97.
4. Lever CJ, Hennessy MS. Adult flat foot deformity. J Orthop Trauma 2016;30(1):41–50.
5. Catanzariti AR, Mendicino RW, Maskill MP. Chapter 46: posterior tibial tendon dysfunction. McGlamry's comprehensive textbook of foot and ankle surgery. 4th edition. Philadelphia: Lippincott Williams & Wilkins; 2012. p. 636–69.
6. Basmajian JV, Stecko G. The role of muscles in arch support of the foot. J Bone Joint Surg Am 1963;45:1184–90.
7. Rodriguez N, Volpe RG. Clinical diagnosis and assessment of the pediatric pes planovalgus deformity. Clin Podiatr Med Surg 2010;27:43–58.
8. Cowell HR, Elener V. Rigid painful flatfoot secondary to tarsal coalition. Clin Orthop Relat Res 1983;177:54–60.
9. Ling SKK, Lui TH. Posterior tibial tendon dysfunction: an overview. Open Orthop J 2017;11:714–23.
10. Henry JK, Shakked R, Ellis SJ. Adult-acquired flatfoot deformity. Foot Ankle Int 2019;4(1):1–17.

11. Kohls-Gatzoulis J, Woods B, Angel JC, et al. The prevalence of symptomatic posterior tibialis tendon dysfunction in women over the age of 40 in England. Foot Ankle Surg 2009;15:75–81.

12. Johnson KA. Tibialis posterior tendon rupture. Clin Orthop Relat Res 1983;177: 140–7.

13. Johnson KA, Strom DE. Tibialis posterior tendon dysfunction. Clin Orthop Relat Res 1989;14(239):196–206.

14. Bluman EM, Title CI, Myerson MS. Posterior tibial tendon rupture: a refined classification system. Foot Ankle Clin N Am 2007;12:233–49.

15. Myerson MS. Adult acquired flatfoot deformity: treatment of dysfunction of the posterior tibial tendon. J Bone Joint Surg Am 1996;78-A(5):780–92.

16. Deland JT, Page A, Sung IH, et al. Posterior tibial tendon insufficiency results at different stages. HSS J 2006;2:157–60.

The Role of Equinus in Flatfoot Deformity

Devrie Stellar, DPM[a],*, Sean R. Lyons, DPM[a,1], Roland Ramdass, DPM[b,c], Andrew J. Meyr, DPM[d]

KEYWORDS

- Pes planovalgus • Triceps surae • Contracture • Calf stretching
- Gastrocnemius recession • Tendo-achilles lengthening
- Posterior tibial tendon dysfunction

KEY POINTS

- Equinus often plays a role in the development of the flatfoot deformity but existing pes planus deformity might also exacerbate equinus.
- Although conservative interventions of equinus do not reverse flatfoot deformity, nonsurgical management of equinus has been shown to improve function and may prevent progression of deformity.
- There are many surgical options for the treatment of equinus and proper procedure selection depends on an accurate diagnosis. Contemporary endoscopic techniques have been developed to potentially reduce wound healing complications.
- Although there is limited literature quantifying the effects of posterior muscle group lengthening on final alignment during flatfoot reconstruction, gastrocnemius recessions and tendo-achilles–lengthening procedures are widely recognized as important adjuvant procedures for adequate correction of pes planus.

INTRODUCTION TO EQUINUS AND FLATFOOT DEFORMITY

Pes planus, otherwise known as flat foot, is a common pathologic condition characterized by a flattened medial longitudinal arch, forefoot abduction, and hindfoot eversion.[1,2] Although ankle equinus and flatfoot are commonly associated, there is some disagreement about whether equinus is the cause or simply the effect of the resulting musculoskeletal deformity. Ankle equinus has been classically defined as any

[a] Inova Fairfax Medical Campus, 3300 Gallows Road, Fairfax, VA 22031, USA; [b] Foot & Ankle Center, P.C., 912 South Pleasant Valley Road, Winchester, VA 22601, USA; [c] Residency Training Committee Inova Fairfax Medical Campus; [d] Department of Podiatric Surgery, Temple University School of Podiatric Medicine, 2nd Floor, 148 North 8th Street, Philadelphia, PA 19107, USA
[1] Present address: 115 West 27th Street, Ship Bottom, NJ 08008.
* Corresponding author. 115 West 27th Street, Ship Bottom, NJ 08008.
E-mail address: devriestellar@gmail.com

Clin Podiatr Med Surg 40 (2023) 247–260
https://doi.org/10.1016/j.cpm.2022.11.002
0891-8422/23/© 2022 Elsevier Inc. All rights reserved.
podiatric.theclinics.com

condition, structural or functional, that limits ankle joint sagittal plane dorsiflexion to less than 10°.[3] Equinus has been associated with more than 30 lower extremity disorders in the literature.[4]

The triceps surae is the most powerful plantar flexor of the ankle joint. The complex consists of the gastrocnemius and soleus muscles within the superficial posterior compartment and their common insertion onto the calcaneal tuberosity via the Achilles tendon after crossing both the ankle and subtalar joints. The gastrocnemius muscle originates from the posterior femoral condyles and thus crosses the knee joint to act additionally as a knee flexor. The soleus muscle originates from the posterior surface of the tibia, fibula, and interosseous membrane and lies deep to the gastrocnemius muscle.[3] The gastrocnemius and soleus muscle bellies converge distally to form an aponeurosis proximal to a common insertion at the Achilles tendon. As the Achilles travels distally, the fibers rotate laterally, resulting in the most medial fibers proximally inserting posteriorly onto the calcaneus.[5,6]

There are numerous potential causes of equinus including congenital structural abnormalities, prolonged nonweight-bearing, poor posture, paralytic conditions, and neurologic impairments.[7] Evolution to bipedal gait has been considered to play a role in the development of equinus because the triceps surae complex must stretch for the heel to purchase the ground.[7] Isolated gastrocnemius equinus is often seen in healthy patients without these predisposing conditions. It is thought that this could be due to the large size of the gastrocnemius muscle and the mechanical advantage that the muscle gains with the knee in full extension.[8]

PATHOMECHANICS OF EQUINUS AND FLATFOOT

Although it is generally accepted that equinus and flatfoot are associated, whether the condition is the cause or the result of flatfoot deformity is still debated.[3,7,9] In normal gait, the subtalar joint pronates from heel strike to midstance. This allows the axes of the midtarsal joint to become parallel and unlock allowing the foot to act as a pronating, mobile adaptor. From midstance to toe-off, the subtalar joint supinates causing the axes of the midtarsal joint to diverge and lock creating a rigid lever for push off. During midstance, the tibia begins to roll anteriorly over the foot leading to the initiation of heel off. Maximum ankle dorsiflexion during gait is required at the initiation of heel off with the minimum required dorsiflexion being 10°.[5]

When ankle equinus is present, the foot does not have the required amount of dorsiflexion to allow for heel off and must be compensated for either proximally or distally. Proximally, ankle equinus can be compensated through lumbar lordosis, hip flexion or genu recurvatum, which brings the center of body mass forward. Although proximal compensation might occur, compensation usually occurs distally within the foot. In the presence of equinus, the subtalar joint will remain relatively pronated causing the midtarsal joint to remain unlocked allowing for increased dorsiflexion at the midfoot. Over time, ligamentous structures begin to stretch, which leads to a progressive flatfoot deformity. As the subtalar joint pronates, the calcaneus everts resulting in the insertion of the Achilles to effectively move to a more lateral position than normal in relation to the subtalar joint. This results in the Achilles being a less powerful supinator, or even a pronator of the subtalar joint in severe cases, which further exacerbates flatfoot deformity.[5]

It has also been theorized that flatfoot might also be a driver to the development of equinus. Medial column incompetence due to ligamentous or tendinous insufficiency results in excessive subtalar joint protonation, which unlocks the midtarsal joint. The increased dorsiflexion leads to increased attenuation of the plantar soft tissues and arch flattening. The talus will remain plantarflexed due to lack of plantar support and the calcaneus will remain everted and declinated resulting in adaptive shortening of the triceps surae complex.[7]

In reality, equinus likely plays a role in both the development of flatfoot and is further exacerbated because of deformity. A tightened triceps surae complex leads to increased force traveling through the midfoot during gait leading to hastened midfoot collapse. Hindfoot collapse also permits greater midfoot flattening and hindfoot eversion resulting in greater adaptive triceps surae tightness.[7]

ASSESSMENT OF EQUINUS IN CONTEXT OF PES PLANUS

Ankle equinus might have different origins and must be assessed clinically to determine the underlying cause of the problem. Classifications of equinus include muscular and osseous. Muscular equinus can be further categorized into gastrocnemius or gastroc-soleus equinus. Isolated soleal contracture in the absence of gastrocnemius pathologic condition has not been specifically identified. Muscular equinus can be further defined as either spastic or nonspastic.

Muscular equinus is most commonly assessed using the Silfverskiold examination where ankle dorsiflexion is measured under the conditions of knee extension and flexion (**Fig. 1**). Limited ankle dorsiflexion with the knee extended but not in a flexed position suggests gastrocnemius equinus. Limited ankle dorsiflexion with the knee extended or flexed suggests gastroc-soleal equinus but might also be due contracture of other posterior structures such as ankle or subtalar joint capsule, peroneal tendons, flexor digitorum longus, flexor hallucis longus, and posterior tibial tendons. In the presence of a flatfoot deformity, the subtalar joint must be corrected out of valgus positioning to neutral or slight varus to accurately measure ankle dorsiflexion. This is only possible in flexible deformities; therefore, it is important to appreciate that the Silfverskiold examination is not reliable in patients with a fixed deformity. To reduce contracture of the ankle extensors and to make the examination more reliable, the examination might be performed in the prone position.[10]

There are several reliable clinical assessment measurement tools that can be used to measure ankle dorsiflexion range of motion during weight-bearing including a goniometer,[11,12] inclinometer,[13–16] or distance to wall tape measurement.[17–19] Konor and colleagues[20] compared the reliability of maximum ankle dorsiflexion range of motion measurements with each of these 3 measurement techniques during stance weight-bearing lunge. Results showed that all 3 techniques had good reliability and low

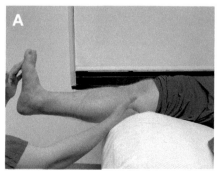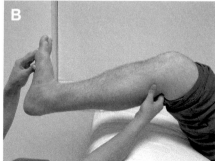

Fig. 1. Silfverskoid test. (*A*) Ankle joint dorsiflexion with knee fully extended. (*B*) Ankle joint dorsiflexion with knee flexed.

measurement error. The inclinometer and distance-to-wall tape measurement techniques yielded higher reliability and lower standard error of measurement when compared with the goniometer technique.[20]

Osseous equinus will present with no change in ankle dorsiflexion regardless of knee extension or flexion. However, compared with gastroc-soleal equinus, osseous equinus will also have a clinically harder end feel during range of motion. Anterior ankle osteophytes and exostoses that may be the cause of an osseous equinus can be assessed with plain radiographs that are obtained during work up of pes planus.[7] Further, a Charger View is a lateral ankle radiographic positioning technique with the patient in maximal ankle dorsiflexion that can further demonstrate osseous impingement as a cause of ankle equinus[21–23] (**Fig. 2**).

As previously mentioned, position of the foot might play a role in the assessment of ankle dorsiflexion with the use of a goniometer as dorsiflexion taking place more distally potentially confounds clinical measurements.[24] In a study by Dayton and colleagues[24] of 50 healthy patients, clinical goniometer measurements of ankle dorsiflexion with the subtalar joint in supination, neutral, and protonation were compared with radiographic measurements of the ankle with the ankle joint in maximal dorsiflexion in each of the 3 rearfoot positions. There was significantly more ankle dorsiflexion recorded using a goniometer when comparing neutral and pronated versus supinated positions. However, radiographic measurements of ankle dorsiflexion showed no corresponding change in each of the 3 foot positions. Thus, radiographs might represent a reliable way to evaluate equinus.

CONSERVATIVE MANAGEMENT OF EQUINUS

Although it is unlikely that conservative care for equinus alone would ever reverse the structural aspects of flatfoot deformity, nonsurgical management of equinus may be beneficial in conjunction with other conservative treatments of pes planus to mitigate further progression. The ultimate goal of equinus treatment is to functionally increase ankle dorsiflexion to facilitate normal gait mechanics. Nonspastic forms of equinus that tend to be seen with flatfoot are usually at least somewhat responsive to conservative measures. A 2013 systematic review and meta-analysis of 23 studies looked at the different interventions for increasing ankle dorsiflexion. Evidence supports static stretching alone, static stretching with ultrasound, diathermy, diathermy and ice, heel raise exercises, and superficial moist heat as forms of treatment.[25]

Manual calf stretching is easy to perform and is one of the most commonly prescribed treatments for equinus. Stretching for just 5 minutes per day for 6 months

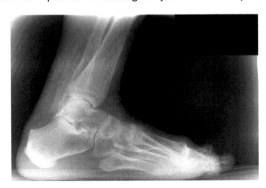

Fig. 2. Charger view. Lateral ankle radiograph with patient in maximal dorsiflexion, evaluating possible osseous equinus.

was found to demonstrate favorable outcomes in a general population by Grady and colleagues.[26] Average ankle dorsiflexion was measured in 25 volunteer medical students after stretching with the knee in extension on one limb. The contralateral, unstretched leg served as the control group. Subjects were randomly assigned a time period of stretching of either 30 seconds, 2 minutes, or 5 minutes per day. Although significant improvements in ankle dorsiflexion was seen in all 3 time periods of stretching, subjects in the 5 minutes per day group showed the greatest improvement in ankle dorsiflexion.[26] Stretching has also been shown to be effective in athletes, with a mean increase of dorsiflexion of 11° seen in a group of runners who underwent an 8-week stretching program.[27]

Stretching exercises can either be performed in a static or cyclic/dynamic fashion, and a 2017 study compared each of these techniques in 20 healthy men.[28] Static stretching consisted of holding maximum ankle dorsiflexion on a footplate for 2 minutes with the hip and knee fully extended. Cyclic stretching consisted of placing the foot on a dynamometer, which would cyclically move the ankle from a plantar-flexed position to 80% of maximum dorsiflexion. Although both groups were found to significantly improve maximum ankle dorsiflexion range of motion, the static stretching group showed a significantly greater response to treatment with average posttreatment maximum ankle dorsiflexion of 29.4° +/− 3.4° compared with the cyclic stretching group of 28.4° +/− 3.5°.[28]

It is thought that effective stretching of the calf muscles is achieved when the foot is adducted, which allows for locking of the subtalar and midtarsal joints through supination.[29] However, more recent literature has shown increased dorsiflexion at the ankle can be achieved with stretching regardless of supination or protonation of the foot.[30,31]

Different techniques for static stretching have been discussed throughout the literature with 2 common techniques including lunging wall stretch and leaning inclined board stretch (**Fig. 3**). Although both have shown efficacy in improvement in ankle dorsiflexion, Kim and colleagues[32] showed that static stretching on an incline board yielded a greater increase in the triceps surae length and ankle dorsiflexion when compared with the lunging wall stretch. Dinh and colleagues[33] further showed that

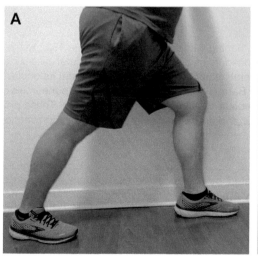
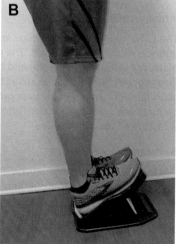

Fig. 3. (*A*) Lunging wall calf stretch. (*B*) Leaning inclined board calf stretch.

gastrocnemius stretching exercises performed in either the weight-bearing or nonweight-bearing positions were equally effective in increasing ankle dorsiflexion.[34]

Botulinum toxin type A is a common treatment of equinus deformity in patients with spastic equinus.[35] Botulinum toxin reduces muscle over activity by reversibly and selectively blocking acetylcholine release at the neuromuscular junction.[36] Botulinum toxin A has been shown to significantly improve passive ankle dorsiflexion and calf spasticity when injected into the medial and lateral heads of the gastrocnemius muscle in stroke patients with spastic equinus at only 1 month posttreatment.[37] The effect of botulinum toxin A at the neuromuscular junction lasts 12 to 16 weeks and repeated injections are necessary in some patients.[38]

Foot orthoses and ankle foot orthoses are a mainstay of conservative management of pes planus. Heel lifts can be placed within orthotics to compensate specifically for equinus. Studies have demonstrated that ankle foot orthoses that limit plantarflexion and provide passive stretching of the posterior calf musculature can reduce progression of equinus deformity in children with cerebral palsy.[39] Foot orthoses might also improve the effectiveness of stretching. In a study examining the effects of standing wall stretching with and without medial arch support, authors found that there was significant increase in the displacement of the gastrocnemius myotendinous junction during stretching in patients who wore arch supports compared with those that did not.[40] Houck and colleagues[41] found that stretching in combination with orthotics has also been shown to significantly improve pain and function in patients with stage II PTTD in a 12-week period in a randomized control trial.

SURGICAL MANAGEMENT OF EQUINUS

Surgical management of equinus consists of posterior soft tissue compartment release. This describes a wide range of procedures that are most commonly performed before distal reconstruction to assist in restoration of the calcaneal inclination angle and reposition the calcaneus inferomedially to support the talus.[1,42] There are numerous approaches to soft tissue release, and this has been classically divided into 3 zones to include the proximal gastrocnemius, gastrocnemius aponeurosis, and the Achilles tendon. Proper procedure selection depends on the patient's physical examination.

Intramuscular Recession

The Silfverskiold gastrocnemius lengthening was originally described in 1924 to treat patients with spastic equinus. The procedure involves a complete proximal gastrocnemius recession of the medial and lateral heads releasing the muscle from its origin.[43] This procedure was later modified by Barouk in 2006 to a release of the aponeurosis of each gastrocnemius head thus protecting the underlying muscle belly.[43] These procedures are considered more historic and are not typically performed in conjunction with flatfoot reconstruction.

Gastrocnemius Recession

Gastrocnemius equinus can be treated by releasing the gastrocnemius tendon or aponeurosis. Recessions at this level are typically performed at the "transection zone," which is located on average 18 mm from the distal aspect of the gastrocnemius muscle belly or 159 mm proximal to the Achilles insertion on the calcaneal tuberosity.[44] Vulpius and Stoffel were the first to describe a distal gastrocnemius tendon inverted "V" recession in 1913.[45] This procedure was originally described with an additional posterior soleus aponeurosis recession that might be appropriate in the setting of gastrocnemius-soleus equinus.[46] In 1956, Baker described a recession of the gastrocnemius tendon as a tongue-in-groove where the distal tongue is sutured back to the proximal tendon in a lengthened position. This suture stabilization might correct for the deformity while preventing the potential complication of overlengthening.[47] This procedure was later modified by Fulp and McGlamry in 1974 where the tongue was created proximally and directed distally.[48] In 1950, Strayer described a transverse release of the gastrocnemius tendon[49] (**Fig. 4**). This procedure is commonly performed in conjunction with flatfoot reconstruction in patients with gastrocnemius equinus because it is relatively easy to perform and can be done in the supine position with a posteromedial incision. Baumann described the release of the anterior aponeurosis of the gastrocnemius muscle belly that allowed the preservation of muscle strength compared with a more distal tendon release.[50] A 2015 cadaveric study compared some of these gastrocnemius techniques and found the Strayer procedure produced significantly greater lengthening and ankle dorsiflexion when compared with the Barouk and Baumann procedures.[51]

Endoscopic techniques have become popular to reduce the possible complications associated with open procedures including wound dehiscence (**Fig. 5**). Similar to the open Strayer gastrocnemius recession, the distal contour of the gastrocnemius muscle belly is used to identify the endoscopic zone. An interval between the gastrocnemius tendon and deep fascia is bluntly dissected and a straight cannula is passed from medial to lateral. An endoscope is passed into the straight cannula and the

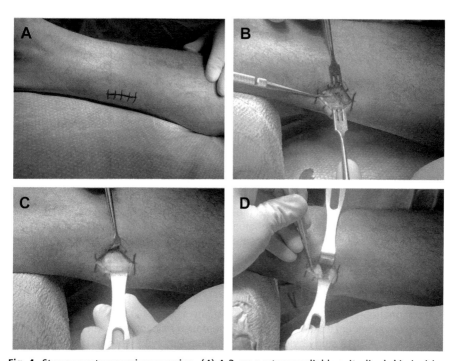

Fig. 4. Strayer gastrocnemius recession. (*A*) A 3-cm posteromedial longitudinal skin incision is made just distal to the gastrocnemius muscle belly and Achilles junction. (*B*) Dissection is then carried through the subcutaneous tissue. The deep fascia is then encountered, which is incised longitudinally. (*C*) Army-Navy retractors are then placed within the deep fascia tissues, ensuring to protect the sural nerve. (*D*) The gastrocnemius tendon is then isolated and complete transection is performed transversely under maximal ankle dorsiflexion.

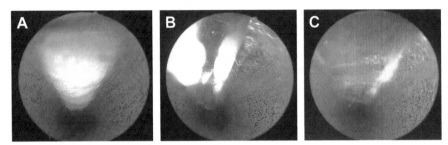

Fig. 5. Endoscopic gastrocnemius recession. (*A*) Identification of the gastrocnemius tendon, ensuring sural nerve is not within the area of transection. (*B*) Hook blade releasing the tendon under direct visualization under maximal ankle dorsiflexion. (*C*) Complete transection of the gastrocnemius tendon is visualized.

gastrocnemius tendon is visualized and examined to avoid the sural nerve during release. The tendon is then resected under direct visualization with the ankle maximally dorsiflexed.[52] The efficacy of endoscopic transection ranges from 83% to 100% in cadaveric models.[52] Mateen and colleagues[53] aimed to better anatomically define this transection zone with MRI as a means to improve the efficacy of this procedure. The transection zone shows an average effective curvature of 126.5° (SD = 6.3°) to which a straight cannula would need to navigate to effectively perform the gastrocnemius recession.[53] In addition they showed an average of 1.2 deep muscular septum (range = 0–2) extending from the aponeurosis at this level.

Achilles Tendon Lengthening

Distal procedures that target the Achilles tendon and are indicated for a combined gastrocnemius and soleus equinus. Numerous Achilles tendon–lengthening procedures have been described in the literature including open Z-plasties to percutaneous hemisections. The Hoke triple hemisection is popular due to ease of technique and the percutaneous nature of the procedure. Introduced in 1931 and modified in 1947 by Hatt and Lamphier, this hemisection is performed at 2.5-cm intervals from the Achilles tendon insertion with the most proximal and distal cuts directed medially and the middle cut directed laterally.[54,55] This triple hemisection has been shown to result in an average increase in ankle dorsiflexion of almost 20°.[56]

A 2017 cadaveric study compared the lengthening effect of 4 different methods of Achilles tendon lengthening.[57] The postoperative maximum degree of dorsiflexion and length of the Achilles tendon were greatest in the rotary triple hemisection and distal double-hemisection groups when compared with the traditional percutaneous triple hemisection. As a result, uneven incision lengthening was seen in this triple hemisection group, whereas the rotary triple hemisection eliminated the Achilles tendon torsion.[57]

Traditional open Z-lengthening procedures are effective in treating equinus deformity; however, recent studies have shown increased efficacy with percutaneous triple hemisection. A 2019 study by Lin and colleagues[58] showed reduced rates of incision complications and reduced risk of equinus recurrence with percutaneous triple hemisection when compared with open Z-lengthening procedure.

Each of these gastrocnemius recessions and tendo-Achilles–lengthening procedures has demonstrated the lengthening ability of the posterior muscle group. Firth and colleagues[59] performed a 2013 cadaveric trial in which they compared the lengthening ability of the procedures described by Baumann, Strayer, Vulpius, Baker, Hoke, and White. They showed the proximal procedures, Baumann and Strayer, were stable procedures but limited in the overall amount of lengthening achieved when compared with the Hoke and White tendo-Achilles–lengthening procedures that produced greater overall lengthening. However, the Hoke and White procedures were neither selective nor stable.[59]

OUTCOMES OF POSTERIOR MUSCLE GROUP LENGTHENING IN FLATFOOT SURGERY

Posterior muscle group lengthening has generally shown excellent results in correction of equinus deformities in conjunction with flatfoot deformities. Rong and colleagues[60] showed significant improvement in ankle dorsiflexion with the knee extended and knee flexed by mean of 13.6° and 9.7°, respectively, in 35 patients who underwent Baumann procedure as part of flatfoot reconstruction with significant improvements seen in functional outcomes scores as well.

Despite the consensus that some release of the triceps surae complex is often required to fully correct flatfoot deformity, there is little literature that quantifies the overall effect that gastrocnemius recession or tendo-Achilles lengthening has on final realignment. This is because it is rarely performed in isolation, and instead represents an adjuvant procedure to other osseous and soft tissue work. In a systematic review of the literature performed by Chang and colleagues[42] in 2020 studying the effects of gastrocnemius recession and tendo-Achilles lengthening on adult acquired flatfoot, the authors found that while there is an overall improvement in range of motion and plantarflexion power as well as radiographic parameters postoperatively, the clinical contribution of posterior group lengthening were hard to separate from concomitant corrective procedures of the foot itself.

Although it might be difficult to fully quantify, posterior muscle group lengthening does seem to play a role in osseous alignment. A recent study in 2021 by Kim and colleagues[61] examined the osseous alignment on preoperative and postoperative radiographs for 97 pediatric patients (150 feet) with pes planus that underwent tendo-Achilles lengthening with coronal Z-plasty for Achilles contracture. Eighty-nine of the 97 patients presented with cerebral palsy. The authors found a significant improvement in Meary's angle and calcaneal inclination angle postoperatively in the idiopathic and cerebral palsy populations. Cicchinelli and colleagues[62] also showed that gastrocnemius recession had a significant effect on the correction of transverse plane deformity in pediatric flatfeet when used as an adjunct to arthroereisis.

COMPLICATIONS OF POSTERIOR MUSCLE GROUP LENGTHENING

Although posterior muscle group lengthening is successful in reducing the equinus deformity, both open Achilles tendon–lengthening and gastrocnemius recession procedures are not benign and might result in complication.[63]

Complications associated with open distal gastrocnemius recession throughout the literature include wound infection/dehiscence, sural nerve injury/entrapment, weakness, atrophy, and cosmetic appearance. Achilles tendon lengthening is more difficult to control with the percutaneous methods and overlengthening is possible, with iatrogenic ruptures reported in the literature.[56,64]

In a series by Rush and colleagues[65] of 126 modified Strayer procedures, 4% of patients complained of dissatisfaction with the incision scar, 3% experienced superficial wound dehiscence or infection, and 2% had sural nerve irritation. There were no complaints of weakness. Similarly, Sammarco and colleagues[66] showed in a series of 40 Vulpius procedures, 5% of patients experienced sural nerve irritation, 25% experienced subjective weakness; however, no reports with dissatisfaction with cosmesis.

They found plantarflexion weakness of the operative limb past 18 months postop when compared with the contralateral nonoperative limb. However, in a series by Duthon and colleagues,[67] they studied patients 1 year after undergoing Strayer procedure for Achilles tendinopathy and showed equal plantarflexion strength when compared with the contralateral limb.

Endoscopic techniques were developed in part to reduce some of these complication rates. These procedures have shown satisfactory results in the correction of equinus. A systematic review including 627 patients found that ankle dorsiflexion improved from −2.3° to 10.9° postoperatively after endoscopic gastrocnemius recession. The overall complication rate was 7.5% with the most common complication being plantarflexion weakness (3.5%), followed by sural nerve injury (3.0%), and wound complications (1.0%).[68] In a study comparing 41 open gastrocnemius recessions compared with 39 endoscopic gastrocnemius recessions authors found an overall 15% complication rate with a significantly greater complication rate using the open technique. Complications in the open group included scar pain, dehiscence/infection, abscess and nerve injury in the open group, whereas only a single case of dehiscence occurred in the endoscopic group.[69]

SUMMARY

Equinus plays an important role in flatfoot deformity. Proper evaluation and surgical management are critical to comprehensively treat and successfully resolved patients' symptoms. We have discussed the cause, evaluation, and some of the common surgical options. Each procedure has its inherent benefits and risks. It is imperative that the foot and ankle surgeons identify and include these procedures as part of the complete reconstructive surgery.

CLINICS CARE POINTS

- Proper evaluation and surgical management of equinus are critical to the cause, evaluation, and surgical options.
- Surgical treatment of equinus has its inherent benefits and risks that must be identified as part of the complete reconstructive surgery for AAFD.

DISCLOSURE

The authors have no commercial or financial disclosures.

REFERENCES

1. Hentges MJ, Moore KR, Catanzariti AR, et al. Procedure selection for the flexible adult acquired flatfoot deformity. Clin Podiatr Med Surg 2014;31(3):363–79.
2. Kaiser P, Guss D. Surgical management of musculotendinous balance in the progressive collapsing foot deformity: the role of peroneal and gastrocnemius contracture. Foot Ankle Clin 2021;26(3):559–75.
3. Meszaros A, Caudell G. The surgical management of equinus in the adult acquired flatfoot. Clin Podiatr Med Surg 2007;24(4):667–viii.
4. DeHeer PA. Equinus and lengthening techniques. Clin Podiatr Med Surg 2017; 34(2):207–27.

5. Aronow MS. Triceps surae contractures associated with posterior tibial tendon dysfunction. Tech Orthopaedics 2000;15:164–73.
6. Pękala PA, Henry BM, Ochała A, et al. The twisted structure of the Achilles tendon unraveled: a detailed quantitative and qualitative anatomical investigation. Scand J Med Sci Sports 2017;27(12):1705–15.
7. DiGiovanni CW, Langer P. The role of isolated gastrocnemius and combined Achilles contractures in the flatfoot. Foot Ankle Clin 2007;12(2):363–viii.
8. Inman VT, Ralston HJ, Todd F. Human walking. Baltimore (MD): Williams and Wilkins; 1981.
9. Root ML, Orien WP, Weed JH. Forces acting upon the foot during locomotion. normal and abnormal function of the foot: clinical biomechanics. Clin Biomech 1977;2.
10. Barouk P, Barouk LS. Clinical diagnosis of gastrocnemius tightness. Foot Ankle Clin 2014;19(4):659–67.
11. Johanson M, Baer J, Hovermale H, et al. Subtalar joint position during gastrocnemius stretching and ankle dorsiflexion range of motion. J Athl Train 2008;43(2):172–8.
12. Norkin CC, White DJ. Measurement of joint motion: a guide to goniometry. Philadelphia: FA Davis Company; 1995.
13. Cosby NL, Hertel J. Relationships between measures of posterior talar glide and ankle dorsiflexion range of motion. Athl Train Sports Health Care 2011;3(2):76–85.
14. Beazell JR, Grindstaff TL, Sauer LD, et al. Effects of a tibiofibular joint manipulation on ankle range of motion and functional outcomes in individuals with chronic ankle instability. J Orthop Sports Phys Ther 2012;42(2):125–34.
15. Denegar CR, Hertel J, Fonseca J. The effect of lateral ankle sprain on dorsiflexion range of motion, posterior talar glide, and joint laxity. J Orthop Sports Phys Ther 2002;32(4):166–73.
16. Grindstaff TL, Beazell JR, Magrum EM, et al. Assessment of ankle dorsiflexion range of motion restriction. Athl Train Sports Health Care 2009;1(1):1–2.
17. Bennell KL, Talbot RC, Wajswelner H, et al. Intra-rater and inter-rater reliability of a weight-bearing lunge measure of ankle dorsiflexion. Aust J Physiother 1998;44(3):175–80.
18. Hoch MC, McKeon PO. Normative range of weight- bearing lunge test performance asymmetry in healthy adults. Man Ther 2011;16(5):516–9.
19. Vicenzino B, Branjerdporn M, Teys P, et al. Initial changes in posterior talar glide and dorsiflexion of the ankle after mobilization with movement in individuals with recurrent ankle sprain. J Orthop Sports Phys Ther 2006;36(7):464–71.
20. Konor MM, Morton S, Eckerson JM, et al. Reliability of three measures of ankle dorsiflexion range of motion. Int J Sports Phys Ther 2012;7(3):279–87.
21. Umans H. Ankle impingement syndromes. Semin Musculoskelet Radiol 2002;6(2):133–9.
22. LiMarzi GM, Khan O, Shah Y, et al. Imaging manifestations of ankle impingement syndromes. Radiol Clin North Am 2018;56(6):893–916.
23. Kingma JJ, Mechielsen J, Cobben LPJ, et al. Radiological assessment of the maximal dorsiflexion position of the ankle in healthy persons. JSM Foot Ankle 2017;2(3):1032.
24. Dayton P, Feilmeier M, Parker K, et al. Experimental comparison of the clinical measurement of ankle joint dorsiflexion and radiographic tibiotalar position. J Foot Ankle Surg 2017;56(5):1036–40.

25. Young R, Nix S, Wholohan A, et al. Interventions for increasing ankle joint dorsiflexion: a systematic review and meta-analysis. J Foot Ankle Res 2013;6(1):46.

26. Grady JF, Saxena A. Effects of stretching the gastrocnemius muscle. J Foot Surg 1991;30(5):465–9.

27. Macklin K, Healy A, Chockalingam N. The effect of calf muscle stretching exercises on ankle joint dorsiflexion and dynamic foot pressures, force and related temporal parameters. Foot 2012;22(1):10–7.

28. Maeda N, Urabe Y, Tsutsumi S, et al. The acute effects of static and cyclic stretching on muscle stiffness and hardness of medial gastrocnemius muscle. J Sports Sci Med 2017;16(4):514–20.

29. Anderson B, Burke ER. Scientific, medical, and practical aspects of stretching. Clin Sports Med 1991;10(1):63–86.

30. Johanson MA, Dearment A, Hines K, et al. The effect of subtalar joint position on dorsiflexion of the ankle/rearfoot versus midfoot/forefoot during gastrocnemius stretching. Foot Ankle Int 2014;35(1):63–70.

31. Johanson MA, Armstrong M, Hopkins C, et al. Gastrocnemius stretching program: more effective in increasing ankle/rear-foot dorsiflexion when subtalar joint positioned in pronation than in supination. J Sport Rehabil 2015;24(3): 307–14.

32. Kim TH, Lim OK, Park KD, et al. Comparison of two static stretching techniques for the triceps surae in healthy individuals: wall and inclined board stretchings. Ann Rehabil Med 2020;44(2):125–30.

33. Dinh NV, Freeman H, Granger J, et al. Calf stretching in non-weight bearing versus weight bearing. Int J Sports Med 2011;32(3):205–10.

34. Jeon IC, Kwon OY, Yi CH, et al. Ankle-dorsiflexion range of motion after ankle self-stretching using a strap. J Athl Train 2015;50(12):1226–32.

35. de Niet M, de Bot ST, van de Warrenburg BP, et al. Functional effects of botulinum toxin type-A treatment and subsequent stretching of spastic calf muscles: a study in patients with hereditary spastic paraplegia. J Rehabil Med 2015;47(2):147–53.

36. Pirazzini M, Azarnia Tehran D, Leka O, et al. On the translocation of botulinum and tetanus neurotoxins across the membrane of acidic intracellular compartments. Biochim Biophys Acta 2016;1858(3):467–74.

37. Picelli A, Filippetti M, Melotti C, et al. Does botulinum toxin treatment affect the ultrasonographic characteristics of post-stroke spastic equinus? a retrospective pilot study. Toxins (Basel). 2020;12(12):797.

38. Friedman A, Diamond M, Johnston MV, et al. Effects of botulinum toxin A on upper limb spasticity in children with cerebral palsy. Am J Phys Med Rehabil 2000; 79(1):53–76.

39. Chen W, Liu X, Pu F, et al. Conservative treatment for equinus deformity in children with cerebral palsy using an adjustable splint-assisted ankle-foot orthosis. Medicine (Baltimore) 2017;96(40):e8186.

40. Jung DY, Koh EK, Kwon OY, et al. Effect of medial arch support on displacement of the myotendinous junction of the gastrocnemius during standing wall stretching. J Orthop Sports Phys Ther 2009;39(12):867–74.

41. Houck J, Neville C, Tome J, et al. Randomized controlled trial comparing orthosis augmented by either stretching or stretching and strengthening for stage ii tibialis posterior tendon dysfunction. Foot Ankle Int 2015;36(9): 1006–16.

42. Chang SH, Abdelatif NMN, Netto CC, et al. The effect of gastrocnemius recession and Tendo-Achilles lengthening on adult acquired flatfoot deformity surgery: a systematic review. J Foot Ankle Surg 2020;59(6):1248–53.
43. Barouk LS, Toullec E, Barouk P. Resultat de la liberation proximale des gastrocnemiens. etude prospective. symposium "Brievete des Gastrocnemiens". Medecine Et Chirurgie Du Pied 2006;22:151.
44. Pinney SJ, Sangeorzan BJ, Hansen ST Jr. Surgical anatomy of the gastrocnemius recession (Strayer procedure). Foot Ankle Int 2004;25(4):247–50.
45. Vulpius O, Stoffel A. Tenotomie der end schnen der mm. gastrocnemius el soleus mittels rutschenlassens nach vulpius. Stuttgart (Germany): Ferdinand Enke; 1913.
46. Takahashi S, Shrestha A. The vulpius procedure for correction of equinus deformity in patients with hemiplegia. J Bone Joint Surg Br 2002;84(7):978–80.
47. Baker LD. A rational approach to the surgical needs of the cerebral palsy patient. J Bone Joint Surg Am 1956;38:313–23.
48. Fulp MJ, McGlamry ED. Gastrocnemius tendon recession: tongue in groove procedure to lengthen gastrocnemius tendon. J Am Podiatry Assoc 1974;64:163–71.
49. Strayer LM Jr. Recession of the gastrocnemius; an operation to relieve spastic contracture of the calf muscles. J Bone Joint Surg Am 1950;32-A(3):671–6.
50. Baumann JU, Koch HG. Ventrale aponeurotische Verlängerung des Musculus gastrocnemius. Oper Orthop Traumatol 1989;1:254–8.
51. Rong K, Li XC, Ge WT, et al. Comparison of the efficacy of three isolated gastrocnemius recession procedures in a cadaveric model of gastrocnemius tightness. Int Orthop 2016 Feb;40(2):417–23.
52. Tashjian RZ, Appel AJ, Banerjee R, et al. Endoscopic gastrocnemius recession: evaluation in a cadaver model. Foot Ankle Int 2003;24(8):607–13.
53. Mateen S, Ali S, Meyr AJ. Surgical anatomy of the endoscopic gastrocnemius recession. J Foot Ankle Surg 2021. S1067-2516(21)00442-00447.
54. Hoke M. An operation for the correction of extremely relaxed flat feet. J Bone Joint Surg Am 1931;13:773–83.
55. Hatt RN, Lamphier TA. Triple hemisection: a simplified pro- cedure for lengthening the Achilles tendon. N Engl J Med 1947;236(5):166–9.
56. Phillips S, Shah A, Staggers JR, et al. Anatomic evaluation of percutaneous achilles tendon lengthening. Foot Ankle Int 2018;39(4):500–5.
57. Chen L, Ma X, Wang X, et al. Comparison of four methods for percutaneous Achilles Tendon lengthening: a cadaveric study. J Foot Ankle Surg 2017;56(2):271–6.
58. Lin Y, Cao J, Zhang C, et al. Modified percutaneous achilles tendon lengthening by triple hemisection for achilles tendon contracture. Biomed Res Int 2019;2019:1491796.
59. Firth GB, McMullan M, Chin T, et al. Lengthening of the gastrocnemius-soleus complex: an anatomical and biomechanical study in human cadavers. J Bone Joint Surg Am 2013;95(16):1489–96.
60. Rong K, Ge WT, Li XC, et al. Mid-term results of intramuscular lengthening of gastrocnemius and/or soleus to correct equinus deformity in flatfoot. Foot Ankle Int 2015;36(10):1223–8.
61. Kim NT, Lee YT, Park MS, et al. Changes in the bony alignment of the foot after tendo-Achilles lengthening in patients with planovalgus deformity. J Orthop Surg Res 2021;16(1):118.
62. Cicchinelli LD, Pascual Huerta J, García Carmona FJ, et al. Analysis of gastrocnemius recession and medial column procedures as adjuncts in arthroereisis for

the correction of pediatric pes planovalgus: a radiographic retrospective study. J Foot Ankle Surg 2008;47(5):385–91.

63. Hsu RY, VanValkenburg S, Tanriover A, et al. Surgical techniques of gastrocnemius lengthening. Foot Ankle Clin 2014;19(4):745–65.

64. Chen L, Greisberg J. Achilles lengthening procedures. Foot Ankle Clin 2009; 14(4):627–37.

65. Rush SM, Ford LA, Hamilton GA. Morbidity associated with high gastrocnemius recession: retrospective review of 126 cases. J Foot Ankle Surg 2006;45(3): 156–60.

66. Sammarco GJ, Bagwe MR, Sammarco VJ, et al. The effects of unilateral gastrocsoleus recession. Foot Ankle Int 2006;27(7):508–11.

67. Duthon VB, Lübbeke A, Duc SR, et al. Noninsertional Achilles tendinopathy treated with gastrocnemius lengthening. Foot Ankle Int 2011;32(4):375–9.

68. Brandão RA, So E, Steriovski J, et al. Outcomes and incidence of complications following endoscopic gastrocnemius recession: a systematic review. Foot Ankle Spec 2021;14(1):55–63.

69. Harris RC 3rd, Strannigan KL, Piraino J. Comparison of the complication incidence in open versus endoscopic gastrocnemius recession: a retrospective medical record review. J Foot Ankle Surg 2018;57(4):747–52.

Single and Double Osteotomies of the Calcaneus for the Treatment of Posterior Tibial Tendon Dysfunction

Jeffrey M. Manway, DPM[a,b,c,d],*

KEYWORDS

- Double calcaneal osteotomy • Lateral column lengthening osteotomy
- Medializing calcaneal osteotomy • Posterior tibial tendon dysfunction

INTRODUCTION

Posterior tibial tendon dysfunction (PTTD) is an increasingly recognized pathologic source of foot and ankle pain. Although the worldwide prevalence of this disorder is not known, studies and surveys suggest that not only is it common for this entity to prompt patients to seek foot and ankle treatment, but significant portions of the population suffer with symptoms of PTTD on a regular basis without seeking medical care. In a phone study by Kohls-Gatzoulis in 2009, 3.3% of female respondents aged older than 40 years were experiencing undiagnosed PTTD with prolonged symptoms.[1] As symptomology has been shown to progress with age, as well as with other confounding factors such as various arthritic conditions and obesity, it is important to improve the understanding of PTTD and potential treatments as the global population expands and is increasingly active at older ages.

The cause of PTTD remains unclear. Although it is clear that ligamentous, osseous and tendinous structures all play a role in the development of symptoms, it is unclear as to the extent of each entity's importance and what underlying factors predispose some patients to developing symptoms while others do not. Further, it is unclear whether entities such as spring ligament attenuation cause PTTD or they are simply downstream effect of the disease. Similarly, it is not well understood whether there is a genetic predisposition to the development of PTTD symptoms. Many efforts have been made to better elucidate pathophysiology of chronic overuse tendon

[a] Chief, Podiatry Section, UPMC Mercy Hospital; [b] Program Director, UPMC Mercy Podiatric Surgical Residency; [c] Clinical Instructor, University of Pittsburgh School of Medicine; [d] Division of Foot and Ankle Surgery, UPP Department of Orthopedic Surgery, 600 Oxford Drive, Suite 200, Monroeville, PA 15146, USA
* University of Pittsburgh School of Medicine.
E-mail address: manwayjm@upmc.edu

Clin Podiatr Med Surg 40 (2023) 261–269
https://doi.org/10.1016/j.cpm.2022.11.007
0891-8422/23/© 2022 Elsevier Inc. All rights reserved.

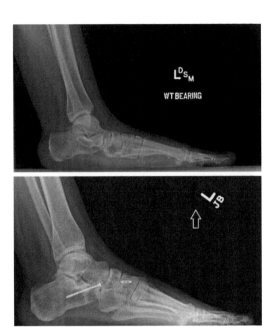

Fig. 1. Preoperative and postoperative images of a 26-year-old woman having undergone an LCL osteotomy, medial cuneiform osteotomy, FDL tendon transfer, and gastrocnemius recession.

injuries and how an antecedent asymptomatic period ultimately leads to permanent tendon degeneration.[2]

PTTD has been classified in stages by various authors with the most commonly used classification being the Johnson and Strom classification.[3] This classification, published in 1989, breaks PTTD into stages 1 through 3, ranging from minimal or no deformity with pain up to rigid, painful hindfoot deformity. This classification, in conjunction with Myerson's addition of stage 4 in 1997, has been used as a guide for providers to dictate surgical treatment.[3] Treatment of PTTD has evolved substantially. Nonsurgical treatment commonly consists of oral anti-inflammatories, injection, activity modification, orthoses, bracing, and physical therapy. Surgical treatment of PTTD has been based on the severity of the disease process and associated arthritis and has substantially evolved from isolated tendon repair historically to now include a

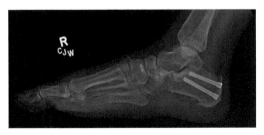

Fig. 2. Postoperative image of a 32-year-old woman having undergone an LCL osteotomy, MCDO osteotomy, medial cuneiform osteotomy, FDL tendon transfer, and gastrocnemius recession.

variety of procedures including joint-sparing osteotomies, tendon repair/transfer, ligament imbrication, or arthrodesis. The ideal patient population and indications for these procedures remain undetermined and outcome studies tend to follow small groups. Specifically, joint-sparing osteotomies have been commonly reserved for patients with stage 2 (flexible hindfoot deformity with pain) PTTD.

Calcaneal osteotomies have shown to be effective adjunctive procedures in the management of PTTD. The difficulty in evaluating their degree of effectiveness, however, lies in the fact that they are virtually never performed in isolation. Rather, calcaneal osteotomies are generally performed in the setting of soft tissue transfers, balancing procedures, or even with arthrodesis. The most commonly studied osteotomies include lateral column lengthening (LCL) osteotomies (Evans/Mosca type) and medializing calcaneal displacement osteotomies (Koutsogiannis type).

Lateral Column Lengthening Osteotomies

LCL osteotomies are commonly used for the management of PTTD (Fig. 1). LCL osteotomies are performed both to modify and correct the overall forefoot abduction, eversion, and dorsiflexion of the foot. LCL osteotomies are considered to be multiplanar corrective procedures. Quite a few iterations of this procedure have been described with the Evans/Mosca types being most commonly referenced in research. Correction of hindfoot valgus has been postulated to be accomplished by mechanisms including direct realignment of the heel, increased tension on plantar ligamentous structures laterally, decreased tension on medial foot structures and adduction of the talus. Lamm and Ernst found that an Evans type LCL osteotomy significantly improved calcaneal inclination angle, tibial-calcaneal angle, tibial calcaneal position, and the antero-posterior talar-first metatarsal angle.[4] The degree of correction has varied among studies and success has either been documented in restoration and maintenance of radiographic values, or in overall patient satisfaction. Ettinger and Plaass evaluated both the Evans (osteotomy between the anterior and middle subtalar facets) and Hintermann (osteotomy between the middle and posterior subtalar facets) LCL osteotomies and found that both procedures significantly improved the talar second metatarsal angle, talonavicular coverage, and naviculocuneiform overlap.[5] There were no statistically significant differences between the 2 groups and both groups also showed significant improvement in FAOS, pain-NRS, and SF-36 scores.

Lateral Column Lengthening Technique

The Evans type LCL osteotomy can be carried out through a typical lateral Ollier incision, modifying this to carry the incision more distally and less proximally. The utility of this incision is that it can be reentered or extended if subtalar fusion is required in the future. Dissection is carried through the soft tissue, retracting the peroneal tendons and sural nerve inferiorly. Dissection should be carried out distal enough to both visualize the calcaneocuboid (CC) joint and permit adequate skin relaxation so as to not lead to iatrogenic nerve, tendon or skin injury during retraction or the osteotomy itself. The osteotomy is classically carried out approximately 1.5 cm proximally to the central aspect of the CC joint, taking care not to penetrate the medial calcaneal cortex. The osteotomy is performed in a vertical fashion, perpendicular to the weight-bearing surface. The author prefers to use a Hintermann distractor with 0.062-inch k-wires to slowly open the osteotomy site. This permits the surgeon the opportunity to progressively open the osteotomy and evaluate the radiographic and clinical degree of correction intraoperatively. The appropriately sized plate, wedge graft or titanium wedge can then be selected and tamped into place. Care should be taken to prevent intra-articular placement of the graft or hardware within the subtalar joint and also to prevent impingement on the peroneal tendons.

Outcomes and Complications

LCL osteotomies have consistently demonstrated the ability to obtain the correction of hindfoot deformity in multiple planes. Frontal, transverse, and sagittal planes all show significant differences in alignment in preoperative and postoperative imaging as measured by tibio-calcaneal, AP talar-first metatarsal angle, and calcaneal inclination angles.[6] Comparing alternative modifications of the technique including osteotomy between the middle and posterior facets, multiplanar radiographic correction has been shown to be significant and modification does not seem to alter the degree of radiographic correction that is achieved.[5] No high-level studies to discern the extent of obtainable radiographic correction exist at this point and careful attention to graft size selection may limit the risks of overcorrection of deformity.

Although it is understood that increasing graft size generally correlates with an increase in degree of correction, optimal graft size is not universally agreed upon. In one titration study, a single millimeter of graft size resulted in 6.8° of correction.[7] Another study looked at strain on the long plantar ligament, finding this reached peak tension at the 6 mm graft size and that greater increase would come at the expense of further strain on the ligament and increased CC joint pressure. Most studies report average graft sizes between 6 and 8 mm although some authors report routinely using 11 to 12 mm graft sizes.[4,7]

Complications of LCL osteotomies, although uncommon overall, include skin breakdown, sural neuritis, peroneal injury, CC and subtalar arthritis, lateral column pain, hardware failure, graft failure, nonunion, and overcorrection. Nonunion has been described in multiple studies. This has ranged from 0% to 15.4%, and a variety of fixation and grafting methods have been studied.[5–11] Allograft has been the most commonly used modality and has not been shown to be inferior to autograft in most studies.[7,10,11] Similarly, porous titanium wedges have been more recently used and not been shown to suffer from increased risk of nonunion or loss of correction.[9] One factor that may ultimately result in nonunion or graft failure is graft size. Particularly allografts greater than 8 mm have been more prone to failure than similar-sized autografts, and increased graft size overall has been associated with poorer outcomes.[7,8]

Loss of correction has been seen as common cause of procedure failure and more recent studies have focused on fixation techniques to prevent graft resorption and failure. In a study by Foster and Hyer, no statistically significant reduction in correction was seen between structural allograft and lateral wedge plating with autograft, although the authors did note a lower nonunion rate in the plate and autograft group.[8] Alternatively, Basile and colleagues evaluated a porous titanium wedge for LCL osteotomy, rather than traditional bone grafting or plating. In their study, they found no instances of nonunion based on absence of hardware loosening and they found no statistically significant loss of reduction in patients after 4-year follow-up.[9]

Hindfoot arthritis and CC joint pressure have both long been viewed as long-term complications of LCL osteotomies. Given the intra-articular nature of the osteotomy, multiple studies have been performed, assessing the safety of osteotomy intervals and outcomes. Similarly, it has been historically hypothesized that increased CC joint pressure results from the procedure, causing lateral column pain. A cadaveric study by Shaer and Cooper found that there was the potential to have excessive load placed on the CC joint with adult Evans osteotomies.[12] However, further studies have shown that early studies may have overcorrected the lateral column and that appropriately sized Evans osteotomies may actually reduce CC joint pressure.[7] Thus, concern about CC joint arthritis may be undue. Differently, development of subtalar arthritis by means of impinging graft or by the osteotomy violating facets themselves are both possible. Multiple studies by Hyer and colleagues have evaluated this problem and have found that the variable nature of the subtalar anatomy makes the reproducible performance of this osteotomy difficult. In one study, they found articular violation and violation of the sustentaculum common, and that the osteotomy should be performed 1.3 mm from the CC joint. Further, erring in a direction of lateral posterior to medial anterior tries to minimize injury.[13]

Medializing Calcaneal Displacement Osteotomies

The medializing calcaneal displacement osteotomy (MCDO), sometimes known as the posterior calcaneal displacement osteotomy, has most commonly been attributed to Koutsogiannis in 1971 but was described as early as 1893 by Gleich.[14] This has been a workhorse procedure in the management of PTTD as an adjunct to posterior tibial tendon repair or flexor digitorum longus (FDL) tendon transfer.

Although the MCDO has been extensively studied, it is difficult to determine the degree of correction and biomechanical effect of this procedure in isolation, given it is almost universally performed in the setting of other concomitant surgeries (ie, FDL tendon transfer, cotton osteotomy, spring ligament repair). In general, the MCDO is not commonly considered to provide multiplanar deformity of the hindfoot. Rather, this is theorized to correct the hindfoot or calcaneal valgus by medializing the heel and thus increasing the supinatory pull of the Achilles tendon. This also has been shown to serve to decrease the lateral contact pressure of the tibiotalar joint and strain at the deltoid over the medial ankle.[14] The MCDO has also been shown to decrease medial foot soft tissue strain and lateralize plantar foot pressure.[15] The optimal degree of correction is not agreed on and may ultimately be patient specific; however, it is understood that both undercorrection and overcorrection can be problematic. In a study by Niki and colleagues, they found that a preoperative lateral talar-first metatarsal angle greater than 25° and a hindfoot tibio-calcaneal angle greater than 15° were both associated with failure of an MCDO and FDL tendon transfer procedure.[15] This may suggest the upper limit of this procedure's effectiveness without further adjuncts. However, there has not been shown to be a strong correlation between the absolute amount of calcaneal displacement and patient-reported outcomes.[15] In an attempt to determine the contribution of the MCDO to overall hindfoot alignment, Ellis and colleagues evaluated a collection of variables. They found that medial cuneiform osteotomy, first tarsometatarsal fusion, spring ligament repair, gender, medial cuneiform position, calcaneal pitch, and MCDO were all statistically significant in their influence on hindfoot alignment. Multivariate analysis isolated the MCDO as the only significant predictor of hindfoot moment arm, underscoring the important contribution of this procedure.[16] Further, the change in degree of hindfoot moment arm seemed to have a linear relationship with the degree of MCDO translation.

Medializing Calcaneal Displacement Osteotomy Technique

The MCDO technique can be carried out in a straightforward fashion. Most commonly performed as an open procedure (although minimal invasive or percutaneous variations have been described), an incision is created posterior to the peroneal tendons and sural nerve and deepened to the level of the lateral calcaneus. It is the author's standard practice to obtain true lateral radiograph to verify the intended osteotomy and incision position. It is important to ensure that the superior aspect of the osteotomy is not exiting too far posterior and also that the inferior aspect of the osteotomy lies distal to the plantar fascial origin. The periosteum is then incised and a lateral to medial osteotomy is created. The obliquity of the osteotomy in both the sagittal and transverse planes can influence the overall degree of hindfoot correction. Once the osteotomy is completed, the tuberosity is medially translated and rotated out of valgus as necessary. It can also be translated inferiorly as to the surgeon's preference. The osteotomy may then be fixated either by screws, staples, or plating.

Complications

Complications of MCDO most commonly include infection, skin healing delay, medial neurovascular injury, sural nerve injury, hardware pain, Achilles tendon injury, undercorrection or overcorrection, and nonunion. Most of these complications can be mitigated by careful surgical technique and thoughtful incision planning and hardware choices. Although direct medial neurovascular injury is more probable, tarsal tunnel syndrome has also been described.[17] Nonunion is a relatively rare complication with multiple studies citing a 0% nonunion rate. Multiple fixation methodologies have been proposed and there does not seem to be a superior option from a union standpoint.[18] However, in evaluating headless versus headed screws, SahraNavard and colleagues found that headed screws were more likely to result in consistent hardware pain.[18]

Double Calcaneal Osteotomies

The term "double calcaneal osteotomy" most typically refers to the combination of an LCL osteotomy and MCDO osteotomy done in the same setting (Fig. 2). As each procedure has distinct advantages, the combination of the osteotomies has been used in an attempt to achieve more comprehensive correction including improvement in both radiographic and functional outcomes. Individually, when compared with one another in conjunction with FDL tendon transfer, patients with an LCL had improved heel inversion relative to the MCDO group while the MCDO group had greater improvement in first ray plantarflexion and varus.[19] Otherwise, both procedures showed comparable improvement in gait speed, pain, stride length, and cadence. As one might expect, the gauge of which procedure is most effective may be attributed to which definition of success is being used. In a meta-analysis by Tao and colleagues, LCL osteotomy, MCDO osteotomy, and triple and double arthrodesis were compared. In this review, optimal outcome seemed driven by the endpoint being evaluated. Lateral talocalcaneal pitch seemed to be best improved by MCDO. Anteroposterior talar-first metatarsal angle and lateral talo-calcaneal angle were best improved by LCL osteotomy. Triple arthrodesis provided the best talonavicular coverage and American Orthopedic Foot and Ankle Hindfoot Score (AOFAS), whereas double arthrodesis provided the best treatment effect on functional scores.[20] In a prospective randomized controlled study by Osman and colleagues, patient outcomes after either MCDO or LCL were collected. Postoperative radiographic measurements were maintained in both groups at 12 months with the LCL osteotomy exhibiting a greater improvement in calcaneal pitch and talonavicular coverage angle.[21]

Together, LCL and MCDO osteotomies have been evaluated in numerous reports. Kou and colleagues evaluated the results of the combination of LCL osteotomy, MCDO, FDL tendon transfer, and gastrocnemius recession. Foot and ankle outcome score (FAOS), ROwan foot pain assessment questionnaire (ROFPAQ), 12 item short form survey (SF-12), and visual analog pain score system (VAS) scores were evaluated. All patients experienced statistically significant improvements in all scoring measurements and scores continued to improve with time, eventually plateauing before 2 years from the date of surgery.[22] In another study looking at midterm results of

LCL, MCDO, FDL transfer and Achilles lengthening, the authors noted a mean AOFAS hindfoot/ankle score of 90 at a mean of 5 years follow-up without any reported non-unions and only a single instance of CC joint arthritis requiring fusion.[23] In another retrospective study, DiDomenico and colleagues evaluated results of a gastrocnemius recession, medial column stabilization, and double calcaneal osteotomy without the use of an FDL tendon transfer. They found at a mean of 14 months postoperatively that there was a statistically significant change in radiologic parameters in structural alignment in this patient population but no validated outcome scoring systems were used.[24] High-level in vivo comparative assessments of single versus double calcaneal osteotomies do not exist. Nunley and colleagues set out to compare different procedure types in a cadaveric model. They compared 6 different combinations of procedures including LCL osteotomy alone (treatment 1), MCDO and FDL transfer (treatment 2), MCDO/FDL Transfer/LCL osteotomy (treatment 3), treatment 3 plus pants over vest spring ligament repair (treatment 4), treatment 3 plus spring ligament repair with the PT tendon stump (treatment 5), and treatment 3 plus spring ligament repair with a suture anchor (treatment 6). Treatments 1 and 3 through 6 all had statistically significant improvements in foot alignment while treatment 2 lost all correction after 1000 simulated loading cycles.[25] The authors also found that inclusion of a spring ligament repair did not significantly alter the exhibited correction.

Double Osteotomy Technique

A double calcaneal osteotomy may be carried out with minimal or no variation regarding the technical performance of the individual procedures. Variations to consider include fixation, incision approach, and degree of correction used when these procedures are performed together. In a series published by Basioni and colleagues, a single-incision approach was used rather than 2 individual incisions. Their study found statistically significant improvements in AOFAS hindfoot scores, lateral AP talo-first metatarsal angles, and lateral talocalcaneal angle. They reported no wound complications and 2 cases of sural neuritis.[26] Although fixation of Evans type osteotomies has not been found to be strictly necessary, numerous fixation techniques have been described in isolation and with double osteotomies. Single screw fixation has been described to fixate both osteotomies simultaneously while avoiding compression of the distal calcaneal allograft.[27]

SUMMARY

Although the publications regarding the utilization of single and double calcaneal osteotomies are voluminous, little consensus exists as to the best practice in performing these procedures. Ample evidence exist to illustrate that single or double calcaneal osteotomies have been shown to be effective in improving patient pain, function and radiographic foot structure. However, no clear, reproducible criteria currently exist to dictate in what environment which combination of osteotomies may be appropriate. Factors such as the desired radiographic criteria to be improved, degree of correction required, planal dominance of the deformity, age and activity level of the patient should all be considered when preparing for surgery.

CLINICS CARE POINTS

- When an LCL osteotomy requires greater than an 8-mm graft size, consider augmentation with a second calcaneal osteotomy or alternative procedure.

- Significant decreases in hardware irritation have been shown with use of headless screws for fixation of MCDO procedures.
- Concomitant spring ligament augmentation does not seem to be an effective adjunct to PTTD surgery in cadaveric studies.

DISCLOSURE

The author has no commercial or financial conflicts to disclose.

REFERENCES

1. Kohls-Gatzoulis J, Woods B, Angel JC, et al. The prevalence of symptomatic posterior tibialis tendon dysfunction in women over the age of 40 in England. Foot Ankle Surg 2009;15(2):75–81. Epub 2008 Oct 1. PMID: 19410173.
2. Guelfi M, Pantalone A, Mirapeix RM, et al. Anatomy, pathophysiology and classification of posterior tibial tendon dysfunction. Eur Rev Med Pharmacol Sci 2017; 21(1):13–9. PMID: 28121362.
3. Abousayed MM, Tartaglione JP, Rosenbaum AJ, et al. Classifications in brief: johnson and strom classification of adult-acquired flatfoot deformity. Clin Orthop Relat Res 2016;474(2):588–93.
4. Lamm BM, Knight J, Ernst JJ. Evans calcaneal osteotomy: assessment of multiplanar correction. J Foot Ankle Surg 2021;S1067-2516(21):00451-8. Epub ahead of print. PMID: 35370052.
5. Ettinger S, Mattinger T, Stukenborg-Colsman C, et al. Outcomes of evans versus hintermann calcaneal lengthening osteotomy for flexible flatfoot. Foot Ankle Int 2019;40(6):661–71. PMID: 30866668.
6. Siddiqui NA, Lamm BM. Digital planning for foot and ankle deformity correction: evans osteotomy. J Foot Ankle Surg 2014;53(6):700–5. Epub 2014 Jun 6. PMID: 24909804.
7. Modha RK, Kilmartin TE. Lateral column lengthening for flexible adult acquired flatfoot: systematic review and meta-analysis. J Foot Ankle Surg 2021;60(6): 1254–69. Epub 2021 Jun 17. PMID: 34253434.
8. Foster JR, McAlister JE, Peterson KS, et al. Union rates and complications of lateral column lengthening using the interposition plating technique: a radiographic and medical record review. J Foot Ankle Surg 2017;56(2):247–51.
9. Matthews M, Cook EA, Cook J, et al. Long-term outcomes of corrective osteotomies using porous titanium wedges for flexible flatfoot deformity correction. J Foot Ankle Surg 2018;57(5):924–30. Epub 2018 Jun 8. PMID: 29891128.
10. Prissel MA, Roukis TS. Incidence of nonunion of the unfixated, isolated evans calcaneal osteotomy: a systematic review. J Foot Ankle Surg 2012;51(3):323–5. Epub 2012 Feb 1. PMID: 22300686.
11. Jara ME. Evans osteotomy complications. Foot Ankle Clin 2017;22(3):573–85. Epub 2017 Jun 13. PMID: 28779808.
12. Bussewitz BW, DeVries JG, Hyer CF. Evans osteotomy and risk to subtalar joint articular facets and sustentaculum tali: a cadaver study. J Foot Ankle Surg 2013;52(5):594–7. Epub 2013 Apr 19. PMID: 23602718.
13. Cooper PS, Nowak MD, Shaer J. Calcaneocuboid joint pressures with lateral column lengthening (Evans) procedure. Foot Ankle Int 1997;18(4):199–205.
14. Peiffer M, Belvedere C, Clockaerts S, et al. Three-dimensional displacement after a medializing calcaneal osteotomy in relation to the osteotomy angle and hindfoot

alignment. Foot Ankle Surg 2020;26(1):78–84. Epub 2018 Dec 7. PMID: 30581061.

15. C Schon L, de Cesar Netto C, Day J, et al, Consensus for the indication of a medializing displacement calcaneal osteotomy in the treatment of progressive collapsing foot deformity. Foot Ankle Int 2020;41(10):1282–5. PMID: 32844661.

16. Chan JY, Williams BR, Nair P, et al. The contribution of medializing calcaneal osteotomy on hindfoot alignment in the reconstruction of the stage II adult acquired flatfoot deformity. Foot Ankle Int 2013;34(2):159–66. PMID: 23413053.

17. Cafruni VM, Bilbao F, Galich F, et al. Tarsal tunnel syndrome following medializing calcaneal osteotomy. Foot Ankle Orthop 2022;7(1). PMID: 35097616; PMCID: PMC8792615.

18. SahraNavard B, Hudson PW, de Cesar Netto C, et al. A comparison of union rates and complications between single screw and double screw fixation of sliding calcaneal osteotomy. Foot Ankle Surg 2019;25(1):84–9. Epub 2017 Sep 6. PMID: 29409301.

19. Marks RM, Long JT, Ness ME, et al. Surgical reconstruction of posterior tibial tendon dysfunction: prospective comparison of flexor digitorum longus substitution combined with lateral column lengthening or medial displacement calcaneal osteotomy. Gait Posture 2009;29(1):17–22. Epub 2008 Jul 7. PMID: 18603429.

20. Tao X, Chen W, Tang K. Surgical procedures for treatment of adult acquired flatfoot deformity: a network meta-analysis. J Orthop Surg Res 2019;14(1):62. PMID: 30791933; PMCID: PMC6385451.

21. Osman AE, El-Gafary KA, Khalifa AA, et al. Medial displacement calcaneal osteotomy versus lateral column lengthening to treat stage II tibialis posterior tendon dysfunction, a prospective randomized controlled study. Foot (Edinb) 2021;47:101798. Epub 2021 Apr 7. PMID: 33957531.

22. Kou JX, Balasubramaniam M, Kippe M, et al. Functional results of posterior tibial tendon reconstruction, calcaneal osteotomy, and gastrocnemius recession. Foot Ankle Int 2012;33(7):602–11.

23. Moseir-LaClair S, Pomeroy G, Manoli A 2nd. Intermediate follow-up on the double osteotomy and tendon transfer procedure for stage II posterior tibial tendon insufficiency. Foot Ankle Int 2001;22(4):283–91.

24. Didomenico L, Stein DY, Wargo-Dorsey M. Treatment of posterior tibial tendon dysfunction without flexor digitorum tendon transfer: a retrospective study of 34 patients. J Foot Ankle Surg 2011;50(3):293–8. Epub 2011 Mar 11. PMID: 21397524.

25. Zanolli DH, Glisson RR, Nunley JA 2nd, et al. Biomechanical assessment of flexible flatfoot correction: comparison of techniques in a cadaver model. J Bone Joint Surg Am 2014;96(6):e45. PMID: 24647512.

26. Basioni Y, El-Ganainy AR, El-Hawary A. Double calcaneal osteotomy and percutaneous tenoplasty for adequate arch restoration in adult flexible flat foot. Int Orthop 2011;35(1):47–51. Epub 2010 Jun 17. PMID: 20556379; PMCID: PMC3014475.

27. Didomenico LA, Haro AA 3rd, Cross DJ. Double calcaneal osteotomy using single, dual-function screw fixation technique. J Foot Ankle Surg 2011;50(6):773–5. Epub 2011 Jul 7. PMID: 21737314.

Addressing Medial Column Instability in Flatfoot Deformity

Scott Schleunes, DPM[a], Alan Catanzariti, DPM[b],*

KEYWORDS

- Medial column instability • Adult acquired flatfoot • Forefoot varus • Talonavicular
- Naviculocunieform • Tarsometatarsal • Cotton

KEY POINTS

- Medial column instability can be directly associated with hypermobility of the medial column and secondarily associated with forefoot supinatus/varus following reduction of hindfoot valgus in stage 2 and Stage 3 Adult Acquired Flatfoot Deformity (AAFD) reconstruction.
- Failure to address medial column instability or forefoot supinatus/varus during AAFD reconstruction can lead to lateral column overload, fifth metatarsal bursitis, as well as strain on the posterior tibial tendon and spring ligament with subsequent recurrence following reconstruction in stage 2 AAFD deformity. In addition, residual medial column instability and forefoot supinatus/varus in stage 3 AAFD can result in strain on the deltoid ligament with subsequent valgus deformity within the tibiotalar joint following hindfoot arthrodesis.
- Surgical management should be considered when forefoot varus deformity is nonreducible, when instability is pronounced, or when degenerative joint disease is present within the medial column articulations.
- The naviculocuneiform joint is less likely to be the primary cause of medial column instability, and in most cases, the primary source of medial column instability is the talonavicular joint.

INTRODUCTION

Adult-acquired flatfoot deformity (AAFD) is a progressive tri-planar deformity characterized by a combination of hindfoot valgus, forefoot varus, abduction of the forefoot on the hindfoot, and collapse of the medial longitudinal arch.[1–4] Johnson and Strom first described a classification for AAFD, which was then modified by both Myerson

[a] Department of Orthopedics, Division of Foot & Ankle Surgery, West Penn Hospital, Pittsburgh, PA, USA; [b] Department of Orthopedic, Allegheny Health Network, West Penn Hospital, Foot and Ankle Institute, 4800 Friendship Avenue N1, Pittsburgh, PA 15224, USA
* Corresponding author.
E-mail address: alan.catanzariti@ahn.org

Clin Podiatr Med Surg 40 (2023) 271–291
https://doi.org/10.1016/j.cpm.2022.11.003
0891-8422/23/© 2022 Elsevier Inc. All rights reserved.
podiatric.theclinics.com

and Bluman[2–4] (**Box 1**). Cotton described the "triangle of support" which showed the normal physiologic foot structure having support from the medial column, lateral column, and heel. He hypothesized that body weight should be transmitted within the confines of the triangle (**Fig. 1**).[5–8] Therefore, deficiency at one location of support will cause ground reactive forces to fall outside the tripod resulting in altered mechanics at the other areas of support. Miller[9] recognized the contribution of medial column instability as it relates to flatfoot deformity and described a procedure that involved arthrodesis of the naviculocuneiform joint (NCJ) with a periosteal flap, first tarsometatarsal joint (TMT) arthrodesis and Achilles tendon lengthening. He reported on 16 patients with satisfactory results and maintenance of the medial arch.[10] Hoke[10] advocated an arthrodesis of the navicular to the first and second cuneiforms along with Achilles tendon lengthening. Since then, there have been various iterations of medial column procedures including joint arthrodesis, medial column osteotomies, as well as medial soft-tissue reconstruction. The medial column is essential in maintaining biomechanical function to the foot in both open and closed kinetic chain. The medial column is made up of both static and dynamic stabilizers, of which injury and/or attenuation can lead to the development of both progressive flatfoot deformity

---

Box 1
Johnson and Strom classification with Myerson and Bluman Modification[2–4]

Stage 1A
    Tenderness along PTT with normal anatomy and normal radiographic findings: secondary to systemic inflammatory disease

Stage 1B
    Tenderness along PTT with normal anatomy and normal radiographic findings

Stage 1C
    Slight hindfoot valgus clinically and radiographically

Stage 2A1
    Supple hindfoot valgus, flexible forefoot varus; radiographic changes include hindfoot valgus, loss of calcanea pitch, Meary line disruption

Stage 2A2
    Supple hindfoot vagus, fixed forefoot varus; radiographic changes include hindfoot valgus, loss of calcanea pitch, Meary line

Stage 2B
    Same as stage 2A2 with addition of forefoot abduction; radiographic changes include talar head uncovering and forefoot abduction

Stage 2C
    Same as stage 2 B with addition of medial column instability, first ray dorsiflexion with hindfoot correction, sinus tarsi pain, radiographic presence of first tarsometatarsal joint plantar gapping

Stage 3A
    Rigid hindfoot valgus, pain in sinus tarsi; radiographically there is loss of subtalar joint space, angle of Gissne sclerosis, hindfoot valgus

Stage 3B
    Same as stage 3A with addition of forefoot abduction

Stage 4A
    Supple tibiotalar valgus

Stage 4B
    Rigid tibiotalar valgus

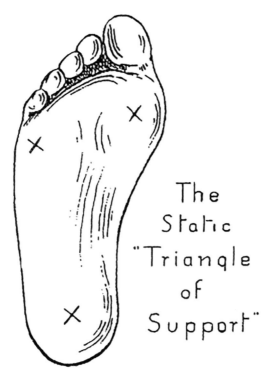

The
Static
"Triangle
of
Support"

Fig. 1. The triangle of support demonstrates the normal physiologic foot structure having support from the medial column, lateral column, and heel.

and hallux valgus deformity. Medial column instability and forefoot varus often result from compensation for hindfoot valgus in AAFD.[11–22] The degree of medial column instability, magnitude of deformity and extent of reducibility, as well the presence of degenerative joint disease (DJD) involving the midfoot articulations and equinus contracture, should be considered when contemplating surgical management. Surgical management of medial column instability generally includes talonavicular joint (TNJ), NCJ, and first TMT arthrodesis, as well as Cotton osteotomy and soft-tissue reconstruction, either performed on an isolated basis or in combination. Medial column instability can be the result of instability at multiple medial column articulations, which can make procedure selection difficult. Open kinetic chain biomechanical examination, dynamic assessment, gait analysis, radiographic findings, intra-articular image-guided injections, and advanced imaging are helpful. However, examination and imaging results will only provide information to help "guide" decision-making and formulate a plan. Fluoroscopic imaging following general anesthesia, as well as intraoperative evaluation and fluoroscopic imaging following hindfoot realignment are also important when considering medial column procedures.

Pathoanatomy

AAFD is defined as a progressive collapse of the medial longitudinal arch with hindfoot valgus, forefoot abduction, and forefoot supination. This progressive collapse of the longitudinal arch can be secondary to excessive subtalar joint protonation, forefoot varus, hypermobility/instability of the medial column, as well as equinus contracture.[1–4] Prolonged collapse of the medial longitudinal arch can lead to forefoot supinatus, which is an acquired soft-tissue adaption in which the medial soft-tissues become contracted. Over the course of time this results in a rigid forefoot supination deformity. As forefoot supinatus progresses, this can be difficult to differentiate from forefoot varus which is a congenital, reducible osseous deformity characterized by a forefoot in varus relative to the rearfoot.[23] Compensatory subtalar joint protonation is necessary to allow the forefoot to be plantigrade in the presence of forefoot varus, which in turn leads to the development of forefoot supinatus and then further subtalar joint compensation, hence the progressive nature of AAFD and its relationship to medial column instability.

The medial column is made up of both static and dynamic stabilizers, and various degrees of frontal plane, sagittal plane, and transverse plane instability can result in pathology.[11–22] Dynamic stabilizers include the posterior tibial tendon and peroneus longus tendon, both with insertions along the medial column. Static stabilizers include the ligamentous structures and plantar fascia. Thordarson and colleagues[24] showed a 25% reduction in medial arch stiffness following complete transection of the plantar aponeurosis. The plantar fascia can also act as a dynamic stabilizer through the windlass mechanism. In a cadaveric study, Rush and colleagues[25] evaluated the effectiveness of the windlass mechanism in regards to transverse positioning of the first metatarsal. They found a 26% increase in first-ray plantar flexion from a deviated first metatarsal position to a corrected position. This may explain the correlation between first-ray hypermobility and the development of hallux valgus. Duchenne[26] was the first to understand the agonist-antagonist relationship between the peroneus longus, tibialis anterior, and tibialis posterior, and postulated that decreased peroneus longus function would inherently lead to elevation of the first ray. Dullaert,[27] in a computed tomography (CT) dynamic cadaveric model, evaluated the influence of the peroneus longus muscle and the positional changes of the TMT, and found that a loaded peroneus longus tendon decreased first-ray instability. In addition, medial column instability along with equinus contracture, inherently increases ground reactive forces to the medial foot with increasing strain on the posterior tibial tendon as well as shortening the level arm of the peroneus longus tendon, adversely affecting its function. This decrease in function of the peroneus longus tendon inhibits its locking ability of the midtarsal joint.[26] The Achilles tendon also acts as the major deforming force with the fulcrum being placed at the mid-foot articulations. Johnson and colleagues[28] in a cadaveric study evaluated the effects of Achilles tendon tension on medial column positioning. They found that as the Achilles load increased, the position of the first metatarsal became significantly more inverted and the influence of the peroneus longus on the medial column became reduced. This increase in medial ground reactive forces can lead to posterior tibial tendon strain and medial column arch collapse at the TNJ. NCJ, first TMT joint, or a combination thereof.

Medial column instability is a key component in AAFD and is often identified following hindfoot realignment in stage 2 and stage 3 AAFD. Failure to address medial column instability or forefoot varus can lead to lateral column overload, fifth metatarsal base bursitis, and strain on the posterior tibial tendon and spring ligament in stage 2 AAFD, as well as strain on the deltoid ligament in stage 3 AAFD. Lateral column overload and fifth metatarsal bursitis are not uncommon following lateral column to lengthen (stage 2 AAFD) and hindfoot arthrodesis (Stage 3 AAFD) when medial column instability or forefoot varus is present. Ground reactive forces will be shifted laterally the following realignment, and an unstable medial column or forefoot varus will result in lateral column overload. Baxter and colleagues[29] in a cadaveric model, evaluated forefoot loading mechanics following lateral column lengthening procedures, and found that overcorrection was directly related to increased lateral column pressures.

Other studies have also shown postoperative lateral column pain following lateral column lengthening in stage 2 AAFD.[30,31] Strain on the posterior tibial tendon and spring ligament can occur when the medial column is unstable in stage 2 AAFD. Medial column instability or residual supinatus/forefoot varus will often lead to elevation of the medial column which requires compensatory subtalar joint protonation for the medial column to purchase the weight-bearing surface. This inherently will place strain along the posterior tibial tendon as well as strain to the spring ligament as the talus plantar-flexes and adducts. In stage 3 AAFD, were compensation of the subtalar joint is no longer available, medial column instability and forefoot supinatus/varus places excess force across the tibiotalar joint with subsequent strain on the deltoid ligament. In some instances, the deltoid ligament is already weakened secondary to prolonged hindfoot deformity. Therefore, compensation for medial column instability will usually take place through the tibiotalar joint leading to the development of tibiotalar valgus or stage 4 AAFD. Miniaci-Coxhead and colleagues[32] evaluated 187 patients who underwent stage 3 flatfoot correction and found that 27% of patients developed tibiotalar valgus at 3.6 months postop. An increase in preoperative Meary's angle was a statistically significant factor associated with development of tibio-talar tilt (**Fig. 2**).

PATIENT EVALUATION

Before any specific assessment of the medial column, it is important to evaluate range of motion of the ankle joint, subtalar joint, and mid-tarsal joint. Ankle joint range of

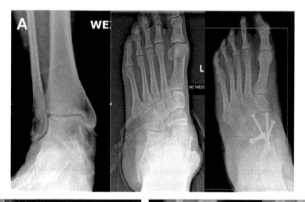

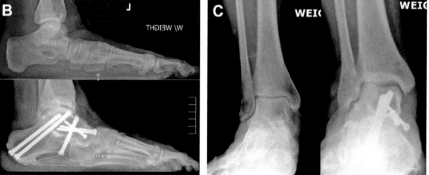

Fig. 2. (A–C): A patient with Stage III adult acquired flatfoot that underwent hindfoot arthrodesis without addressing residual forefoot varus. This patient developed tibiotalar valgus approximately within 1 year following surgery.

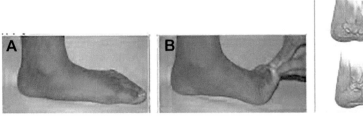

Fig. 3. The Hubschner Maneuver can be utilized to assess the reducibility of the medial longitudinal arch and rear foot through the Windlass Mechanism (figure A–C).

motion should be assessed with both the knee in an extended position and flexed position while the mid-tarsal joint is in a locked position to quantify the extent and type of equinus. Evaluation of tritarsal range of motion is important to determine the reducibility of the hindfoot deformity. Both double heel rise and the hallux raise maneuvers can be used to further determine the reducibility of the hindfoot valgus and longitudinal arch collapse, and single heel rise can help ascertain the functionality of the posterior tibial tendon (**Figs. 3**A–C and **4**). Palpation of the navicular tuberosity, posterior tibial tendon, deltoid ligament, sinus tarsi, and sub-fibular regions are also important in determining which anatomic structures are contributing to the patient's symptom complex.

A focused examination specifically evaluating the forefoot-to-hindfoot relationship as well as assessing first-ray hypermobility are important. Forefoot to hindfoot relationship should be assessed with the foot placed in neutral position by centering the navicular on the head of the talus. As the hindfoot is held in position with one hand, the opposite hand is used to passively bring the ankle to neutral dorsiflexion by placing force on the plantar aspect of the fourth and fifth metatarsal heads. The relationship of the first and fifth metatarsals are evaluated by viewing the foot "head on". This can be seen in **Fig. 5** which shows a skeletal model of forefoot varus and **Fig. 6** which shows a physical examination of a patient with forefoot varus deformity (see **Figs. 5** and **6**). It is essential not only to identify forefoot varus, but to also determine the degree of reducibility. To assess stability of the first ray, the patient should be placed in a seated position and the lesser metatarsals should be stabilized with one hand, whereas the opposite hand is used to manipulate the first metatarsal.

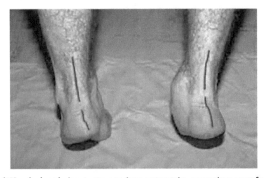

Fig. 4. Double and Single heel rise tests are important in assessing rearfoot reducibility and assessing posterior tibial tendon strength.

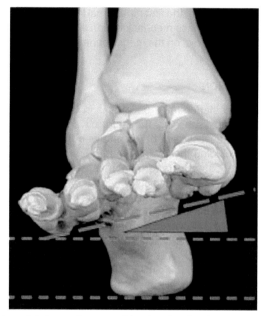

Fig. 5. This skeletal model shows the neutral heel with a forefoot that in in varus relative to the rearfoot consistent with forefoot varus.

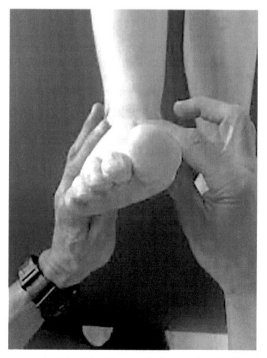

Fig. 6. Forefoot varus can be identified in physical exam by placing the subtalar joint in neutral and comparing the neutral calcaneal stance position to the forefoot position.

Dorsiflexion and plantarflexion of the first metatarsal in relation to the medial cuneiform should be assessed. The windlass mechanism can also be engaged to assess dorsal subluxation of the first metatarsal on the medial cuneiform. One should also assess for joint crepitus and pain.[23]

RADIOGRAPHIC EVALUATION

Weight-bearing anteroposterior (AP), oblique, and lateral radiographs of the foot play an important role in assessing the deformity. Lateral weight-bearing radiographs provide the best assessment of the medial column. It is important to assess each individual joint, including the TNJ, NCJ, and first TMT joint. Asymmetrical joint space narrowing, dorsal osteophyte formation as well as periarticular sclerosis can be indicative of medial column instability. In addition, the degree of angular deformity should be noted. An increase in Meary's angle can be indicative of medial column instability, and by identifying the apex of the deformity, one can determine the location(s) of instability. A calcaneal pitch angle less than 19° has been shown to provide the best assessment of injury to supporting medial column structures, including the deltoid ligament.[33] A "sag" can be visualized as a depression along the medial column and can be indicative of joint instability. This can take place at a single joint, or at multiple joints along the medial column. Medial column elevation is best evaluated on a lateral weight-bearing radiograph by assessing the relationship between the first and second metatarsal in the sagittal plane. The Seiberg's index can be useful in evaluating first metatarsal elevation. The Seiberg's index is defined as the difference between the perpendicular distance in millimeters, from the dorsal aspect of the first metatarsal shaft to the dorsal aspect of the second metatarsal shaft at the neck of the first metatarsal and 15 mm from the base. The value at the base is then subtracted from the value at the metatarsal neck. A value greater than 1 mm is indicative of first ray elevation.[34] Medial column elevation can be indicative of residual forefoot supinatus, uncompensated forefoot varus, or hypermobility along the medial column. **Fig. 7** is a lateral weight-bearing radiograph that shows significant first ray elevation consistent with forefoot varus and medial column instability (see **Fig. 7**). Assessing radiographs for DJD as well as location/apex of deformity can be helpful with surgical planning. Intraoperative fluoroscopy is helpful to assess the medial column position following hindfoot realignment; however, intraoperative simulation of weight bearing is not always reliable. Weightbearing CT scans can also be helpful in better assessing medial column position and joint degeneration.

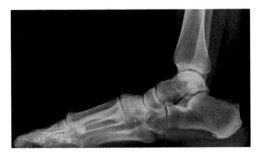

Fig. 7. This figure demonstrates a lateral weight bearing radiograph with elevation of the medial column consistent with medial column instability. The dorsal cortex of the first metatarsal is elevated relative to the cortex of the second metatarsal.

SURGICAL DECISION-MAKING

Surgical management of medial column instability can include arthrodesis of the TNJ, NCJ, and/or the first TMT joint, as well as first cuneiform osteotomy. Procedure selection should be based on degree and reducibility of hindfoot deformity, degree and reducibility of forefoot varus following hindfoot realignment, the laxity of soft-tissues, the presence of DJD, as well as the presence of equinus. The decision to proceed with medial column stabilization is often made intraoperatively, following hindfoot realignment. Assessing the degree and flexibility of AAFD is important when considering procedures to address medial column instability and forefoot varus. Reducibility of hindfoot valgus can be determined with a double heel rise, as well as with open kinetic chain evaluation. The reducibility of longitudinal arch collapse can be determined with a hallux raise test. In general, medial column stabilization in stage II AAFD can be addressed with TNJ-sparing procedures including NCJ and first TMT joint arthrodesis as well as with a Cotton osteotomy. However, TNJ arthrodesis is often indicated in non-reducible stage 3 or 4 AAFD. There are exceptions in which a patient with a reducible AAFD may benefit from TNJ arthrodeisis. These exceptions include patients with severe deformity, soft-tissue adaption, degenerative changes to the tri-tarsal complex, severe medial column instability that will unlikely respond to periarticular osteotomies, and patients with pronounced soft-tissue laxity, that is, Ehlers-Danlos syndrome. Stage 2 procedures may also be used in conjunction with hindfoot arthrodesis in patients with gross instability or in those with residual forefoot varus following hindfoot arthrodesis. The optimal level of medial column stabilization will vary depending on the aforementioned factors.

Naviculocuneiform Arthrodesis

NCJ arthrodesis is a versatile procedure that can be used in stage 2 AAFD to address medial column instability and severe forefoot varus (**Fig. 8**) NCJ arthrodesis can also be used concomitantly with TNJ arthrodesis in stage 3 and stage 4 AAFD to impart medial column stability and restore the forefoot-to-hindfoot frontal plane relationship, especially in patients with significant residual forefoot abduction and forefoot supinatus/varus not fully reduced with TNJ arthrodesis (**Fig. 9A–C**). Lungren and colleagues[35] evaluated *in vivo* range of motion of the NC joint in six patients, and found that the average range of motion was 11.5°, 10.4°, and 6.2° in the sagittal plane, frontal plane, and transverse plane, respectively. This joint showed range of motion similar to the talocalcaneal articulation. Medial column instability at the level of the NC joint can also manifest as DJD and sometimes present as an NC fault or sag on a lateral weight bearing radiograph. However, this is highly variable. **Fig. 9A–C**, courtesy of Metzl and colleagues[36] showed naviculocunieform sag on a lateral weight-bearing radiograph (**Fig. 10A, B**). NCJ arthrodesis in this situation can impart stability of the medial column and restore the forefoot-to-hindfoot frontal plane relationship. Arthrodesis rates of the NCJ are relatively high. Ajis and colleagues[37] had a 97% fusion rate in 20 patients who underwent NC fusion for symptomatic flatfoot. Secondarily, there was also a significant improvement of both Meary's angle and talar head coverage following isolated NC fusion. Given these findings along with the relatively low complication rate, arthrodesis of the NCJ in stage 3 AAFD, while sparing the TNJ, has shown to be beneficial. Studies have shown that arthrodesis of the TNJ significantly limits hindfoot motion and can accelerate arthritic changes to neighboring joints.[38] Steiner and colleagues[39] proposed combined STJ and NC arthrodesis in the treatment of stage 3 rigid flat foot to preserve the TNJ as a mobile adapter. Their cohort involved 31 patients with 34 feet who underwent combined STJ and NC fusion.

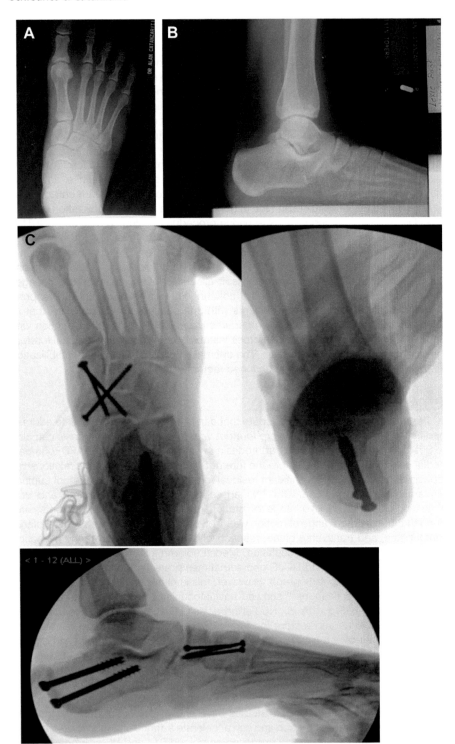

Fig. 8. (A–C): This is a patient with stage II adult acquired flatfoot as well as medial column instability. This patient underwent naviculocuneiform arthrodesis as well as a medial displacement calcaneal osteotomy.

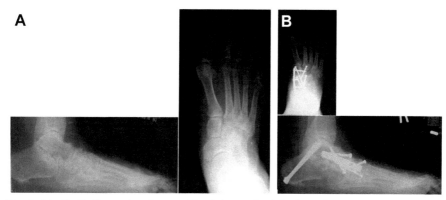

Fig. 9. (*A, B*): Radiographs of stage III adult acquired flatfoot that underwent hindfoot arthrodesis as well as naviculocuneiform arthrodesis to address residual forefoot varus following hindfoot realignment.

Fifteen patients also required a concomitant medial displacement calcaneal osteotomy for further correction. Radiographically, they found significant correction in Meary's angle, TNJ coverage angle, and Simmons angle. They reported one nonunion at the STJ and one nonunion at the NCJ, as well as one patient who required total ankle arthroplasty secondary to lateral talar AVN. They concluded that this was a safe and powerful combination that resulted in good results and a significant decrease in peritalar subluxation.[39,40] Sparing the TNJ might also prevent the development of early ankle arthritis as well as tibiotalar valgus following hindfoot arthrodesis.

Medial Cuneiform Osteotomy: Cotton Osteotomy

The medial cuneiform osteotomy, also known as the Cotton osteotomy can be used to address medial column instability and forefoot varus/supinatus in both stage 2 AAFD and stage 3/4 AAFD. This is an opening wedge osteotomy performed in the mid substance of the medial cuneiform (**Fig. 11**). The cotton osteotomy functions much like the NCJ arthrodesis, providing medial column stability and structural realignment in the sagittal plane (**Fig. 12A–E**). Although this osteotomy does not have the same power or capacity of an NCJ arthrodesis; however, there are some advantages. A Cotton

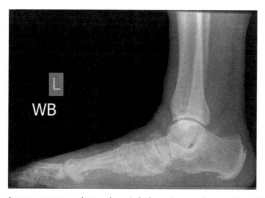

Fig. 10. This figure demonstrates a lateral weightbearing radiograph with a fault a the level of the navicular- cuneiform Joint.

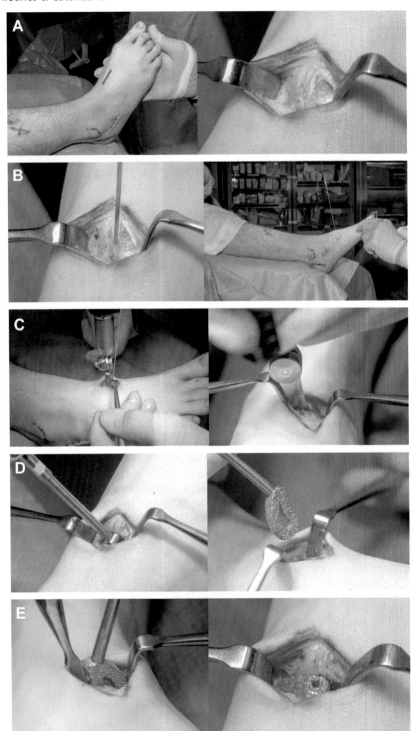

Fig. 11. (*A–E*) Cotton osteotomy. This osteotomy is performed at the mid substance of the medial cuneiform. The authors use a Kirschner wire to provide sagittal plane orientation. This osteotomy should be perpendicular to the bone so that the distal articulation is not invaded with the saw.

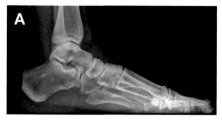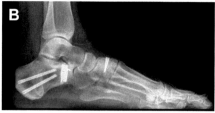

Fig. 12. (A, B) Cotton osteotomy. Radiographs demonstrating a cotton osteotomy as well as several other ancillary procedures, for correction of stage II adult acquired flatfoot. A metal wedge was utilized to obtain sagittal plane correction.

osteotomy can have a protective effect on the NC and first TMT articulations by maintaining residual motion along the medial column. In addition, the Cotton osteotomy can further enhance stability by engaging the windlass mechanism through plantar-flexion of the first ray. The Cotton osteotomy is an effective ancillary procedure to address forefoot varus following hindfoot arthrodesis in stage 3 and stage 4 AAFD (**Fig. 13**A, B) Residual forefoot varus following rearfoot arthrodesis can lead to major complications including failed arthrodesis as well as tibiotalar valgus deformity. Southwell and colleagues[30] found that 11% of failed triple arthrodesis occurred as a direct result of residual forefoot varus deformity. Vacketta and colleagues[7] reviewed 47 consecutive patients who underwent hindfoot arthrodesis for stage 3 AAFD, comparing 25 patients with an adjunct Cotton osteotomy with 27 patients in a control group, without osteotomy. Eight of the nine patients who developed tibiotalar valgus on follow-up AP radiographs of the ankle did not have a cotton osteotomy, demonstrating the protective effect of the Cotton osteotomy on the medial soft-tissue structures supporting the tibiotalar articulation.

Scott and colleagues,[41] in a cadaveric study, found that every millimeter of graft size will contribute 1.9° of plantar flexion to the first ray, but the ideal amount of optimal correction has not been established. In a similar radiographic study, Kunas and colleagues[42] found significant correction in calcaneal inclination angle, with each millimeter change in graft size, correlating with a 2.1° increase in the calcaneal inclination angle. The authors also use this osteotomy in surgical management of adolescent flatfoot deformity. We will consider a Cotton osteotomy for residual forefoot supinatus/varus following lateral column lengthening or subtalar arthroereisis. This osteotomy avoids the growth plates and eliminates the problems associated with arthrodesis in the pediatric population. **Fig. 14**A, B shows a pediatric patient who underwent flexible flatfoot reconstruction with arthroereisis with residual forefoot varus that was corrected with a Cotton osteotomy (see **Fig. 14**A, B). In general, the Cotton osteotomy provides stability and sagittal plane realignment to the medial column, to a lesser extent than NCJ arthrodesis, but is a joint sparing option with fewer complications.

First Tarsometatarsal Arthrodesis

first TMT joint arthrodesis is another surgical option in the treatment of medial column instability. Surgical indications for first TMT joint arthrodesis include gross instability or hypermobility, degenerative changes contributing to the symptom complex, concomitant hallux valgus deformity, or when the apex of the deformity is at the first TMT joint. Hypermobility of the first ray is a common finding in patients with stage 2 or 3 flatfoot deformity as well as severe hallux valgus deformity. Previous studies have shown that

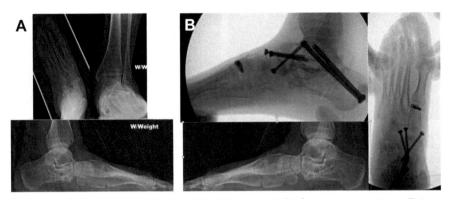

Fig. 13. (*A, B*): Radiographs of a stage III adult acquired flatfoot reconstruction utilizing a cotton osteotomy to address residual forefoot varus.

normal first TMT range of motion is approximately 10° in the sagittal position with neutral position being zero degrees.[43] Those patients with an increased range of motion in the dorsal direction are considered to have a hypermobile first ray. As the first ray elevates, the subtalar joint is forced to pronate to compensate for this elevation, and the hallux abducts and rotates in a valgus direction to purchase the ground and prevent jamming of the first metatarsophalangeal joint. In a biomechanical study, Cowie and colleagues[44] compared first TMT range of motion of control patients with patients who had flatfoot deformity and associated first TMT arthritis. They found a significant increase in TMT range of motion in the latter cohort and stated that first TMT hypermobility may lead to progression of flatfoot deformity. They concluded that first TMT joint arthrodesis is a reasonable consideration for flatfoot correction when hypermobility is present. Johnson and colleagues[45] evaluated the effects of isolated first TMT arthrodesis on hindfoot alignment radiographic measurements and found significant changes in talar declination, lateral talocalcaneal angle, Meary's angle, medial cuneiform height, talocalcaneal angle, and talar head coverage. Day and colleagues[46] evaluated the contribution of first TMT joint arthrodesis in the treatment of stage 3 AAFD with concomitant subtalar joint arthrodesis and found that there was

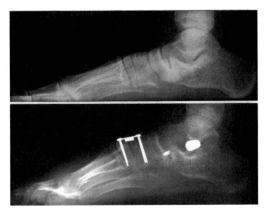

Fig. 14. This figure demonstrates a pediatric patient who underwent flexibile flatfoot reconstruction with arthroereisis with residual forefoot varus that was corrected with a cotton osteotomy.

correction in all radiographic parameters except for calcaneal pitch, but more importantly found that there was no change or worsening of NC joint deformity at follow-up. Residual forefoot varus or supinatus with the apex at the first TMT joint, can also be corrected with arthrodesis.

First ray shortening and elevation, with associated hypermobility, is associated with Myerson stage 2-d AAFD.[47] (**Fig. 15**) and (**Fig. 16**) represent a patients who presented with stage 2-d AAFD with associated first TMT joint hypermobility, as well as first ray shortening and elevation. This flatfoot is driven by first ray insufficiency. As such, all components of first ray insufficiency should be addressed. Surgical goals were to avoid further shortening, restore sagittal plane alignment and reduce medial column instability.

In summary, The first TMTJ arthrodesis has been shown to be an option for the treatment of medial column instability in the presence of first TMT joint hypermobility, degenerative changes, hallux valgus deformity, and when the apex of deformity is located at the first TMT joint.

Talonavicular Arthrodesis

Talonavicular arthrodesis is the most powerful procedure in the treatment of medial column instability and is generally reserved for stage 3 or stage 4 flatfoot deformities. In general, medial column instability is likely secondary to the TNJ, even when the apex of the deformity appears to be distal. The TNJ provides the majority of compensatory motion to the hindfoot, and as the talus adducts and plantarflexes relative to the navicular, stresses are increased along the medial column. Studies have shown that arthrodesis of the TNJ significantly decreases motion at the subtalar joint and calcaneocuboid joint, which further provides stability to the hindfoot.[38] Due to the relative decrease in compensatory motion in the hindfoot following TNJ arthrodesis,

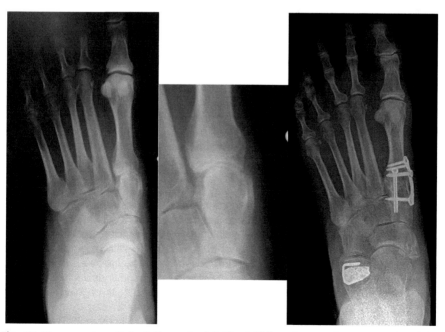

Fig. 15. Myerson stage 2-d adult acquired flatfoot. This patient underwent 1st TMT joint arthrodesis as well as lateral column lengthening.

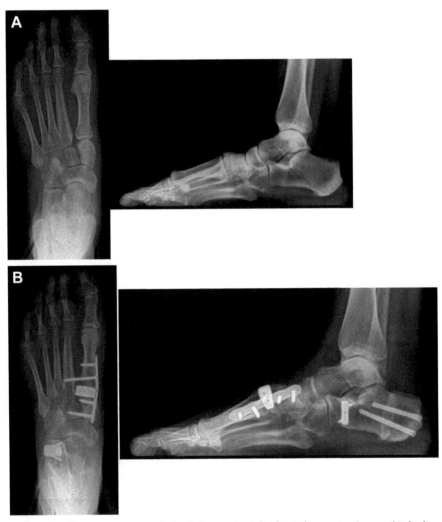

Fig. 16. (*A, B*): Myerson stage 2-d adult acquired flatfoot demonstrating sagittal plane realignment following TMT arthrodesis with metal spacer as well as lateral column lengthening.

concomitant medial column procedures may be indicated to correct residual forefoot supinatus/varus following hindfoot realignment. Although TNJ arthrodesis is generally avoided in patients with reducible flatfoot deformity, there is a subset of patients with gross instability or ligamentous laxity in which extra-articular osteotomies are inadequate. Deformity in these patients cannot be fully reduced with osteotomies due to insufficient soft-tissue constraints. TN arthrodesis might be indicated in this group of patients (**Fig. 17**A, B). This is also true in patients with conditions such as Marfan's disease and Ehlor's Danlos syndrome, who continue to pronate through any corrective osteotomies. The Beighton hypermobility score assessment, can be beneficial in determining the presence of any hypermobility syndrome.[48] In general, TNJ arthrodesis is a powerful procedure in stage 3 and stage 4 AAFD, but one must be cognizant of both forefoot and hindfoot position, as degernative changes can develop at

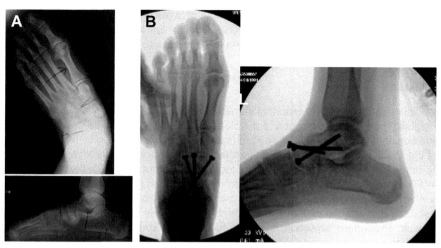

Fig. 17. (*A, B*): Stage II adult acquired flatfoot with grossly unstable hindfoot valgus and medial column instability. We chose to proceed with TN arthrodesis.

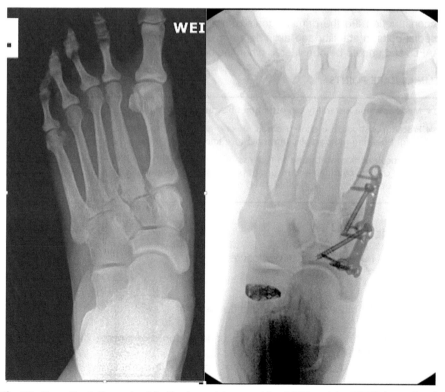

Fig. 18. Stage II adult acquired flatfoot requiring combined NCJ and 1st TMT joint arthrodesis to address severe deformity as well as pronounced instability.

neighboring joints given the loss of compensation at the tri-tarsal complex. Harper and colleagues[49] reviewed 27 patients who underwent isolated TNJ arthrodesis and found 5 (18.5%) patients developed degenerative changes to neighboring joints, but all maintained alignment.

SUMMARY

Medial column stability is essential in maintaining normal mechanics during gait and instability can lead to progressive development of AAFD as well as hallux valgus. In addition, instability of the medial column can be directly associated with hypermobility of the medial column articulations. Furthermore, forefoot supinatus/varus is not uncommon following the reduction of hindfoot valgus deformity in both flexible and fixed AAFD reconstruction. The authors recommend considering medial column stabilization and realignment as a component part of AAFD reconstruction. Medial column instability can oftentimes be multi-factorial, which makes the selection of procedures difficult. Procedure selection is often challenging. Procedures should be chosen based on open and closed kinetic chain preoperative physical examination, weight-bearing radiographs, intraoperative imaging and intraoperative examination. The authors prefer to avoid arthrodesis of two adjacent joints to decrease medial column rigidity and progression of neighboring joint arthritis. Nonetheless, all articulations contributing to the instability or deformity should be included (**Fig. 18**A, B). Preventing lateral column overload and recurrent posterior tibial tendon dysfunction with subsequent deformity in flexible AAFD reconstruction, as well as preventing valgus deformity with subsequent degeneration of the tibiotalar joint in rigid AAFD reconstruction are the primary goals of medial column stabilization. Restoration of medial column stability and alignment are essential in the surgical management of AAFD, and should be considered when indicated.

CLINICS CARE POINTS

- Medial column instability can oftentimes be multi-factorial.
- Procedures should be chosen based on gait analysis, preoperative physical examination, weight-bearing radiographs, intraoperative imaging and intraoperative examination.
- All articulations contributing to the instability or deformity should be included to prevent lateral column overload and recurrent posterior tibial tendon dysfunction with subsequent deformity in flexible AAFD reconstruction.

DISCLOSURE

The authors have no financial disclosures.

REFERENCES

1. Deland JT. MD adult-acquired flatfoot deformity. J Am Acad Orthop Surg 2008; 16(7):399–406.
2. Johnson KA, Strom DE. Tibialis posterior tendon dysfunction. Clin Orthop Relat Res 1989;239:196–206.
3. Myerson MS. Adult Acquired Flatfoot Deformity: treatment of dysfunction of the posterior tibial tendon. JBJS Am 1996;78:780–92.
4. Bluman EM, Title CI, Myerson MS. Posterior tibial tendon rupture: a refined classification system. Foot Ankle Clin 2007;12:233–49.

5. Cotton FJ. "Foot statics and surgery". N Engl J Med 1936;214(8):353–62.
6. Hirose CB, Johnson JE. Plantarflexion opening wedge medial cuneiform osteotomy for correction of fixed forefoot varus associated with flatfoot deformity. Foot Ankle Int 2004;25(8):568–74.
7. Vincent Vacketta G, Jones Jacob M, Catanzariti Alan R. Radiographic analysis and clinical efficacy of hindfoot arthrodesis with versus without cotton osteotomy in stage iii adult acquired flatfoot Deformity. J Foot Ankle Surg 2021;61(4):879–85.
8. Lutz M, Myerson M. Radiographic analysis of an opening wedge osteotomy of the medial cuneiform. Foot Ankle Int 2011;32(3):278–87.
9. Miller OL. A plastic flat foot operation. J Bone Joint Surg 1927;9 -(1):84–91T.
10. Jeffrey Boberg S, McMurray Sean J. Evaluation of the medial column in flatfoot surgery. Clin Podiatr Med Surg 2007;24(Issue 4):721–33. ISSN 0891-8422.
11. Lui. Stabilization of medial longitudinal foot arch by peroneus longus transfer. Foot 2016;27:22–6.
12. Huang C-K, Kitaoka HB, An K-N, et al. Biomechanical evaluation of longitudinal arch stability. Foot & Ankle. 1993;14(6):353–7.
13. Rachel Lucas, Cornwall Mark. Influence of foot posture on the functioning of the windlass mechanism. Foot 2017;30:38–42.
14. Pomeroy GC, Pike RH, Beals TC, et al. Acquired flatfoot in adults due to dysfunction of the posterior tibial tendon. J Bone Joint Surg Am 1999;81:1173–82.
15. Chi TD, Toolan BC, Sangeorzan BJ, et al. The lateral column lengthening and medial column stabilization procedures. Clin Orthop 1999;365:81–90.
16. DiGiovanni CW, Langer P. The role of isolated gastrocnemius and combined Achilles contractures in the flatfoot. Foot Ankle Clin 2007;12:363–79.
17. Myerson MS, Badekas A, Schon LC. Treatment of stage II posterior tibial tendon deficiency with flexor digitorum longus tendon transfer and calcaneal osteotomy. Foot Ankle Int 2004;25:445–50.
18. Rush SM, Jordan T. Naviculocuneiform arthrodesis for treatment of medial column instability associated with lateral peritalar subluxation. Clin Podiatr Med Surg 2009;26(Issue 3):373–84.
19. Kadakia AR, Kelikian AS, Barbosa M, et al. Did failure occur because of medial column instability that was not recognized, or did it develop after surgery? Foot Ankle Clin 2017;22(3):545–62.
20. Gross CE, Jackson JB 3rd. The importance of the medial column in progressive collapsing foot deformity: osteotomies and stabilization. Foot Ankle Clin 2021;26:507–21.
21. Smith JT, Bluman EM. Update on stage IV acquired adult flatfoot disorder: when the deltoid ligament becomes dysfunctional. Foot Ankle Clin 2012;17(2):351–60.
22. Blackwood Steven, Gossett Leland. Hallux valgus/medial column instability and their relationship with posterior tibial tendon dysfunction. Foot Ankle Clin 2018; 23(2):297–313.
23. Evans Erica L, Catanzariti Alan R. Forefoot supinatus. Clin Podiatr Med Surg 2014;31(3):405–13.
24. Thordarson DB, Schm O, et al. J. Dynami c support of the human longitudinal arch. A biomechanical evaluation. Clin Orthop 1995;316:165–72.
25. Rush Shannon M, Christensen Jeffrey C, Johnson Cherie H. Biomechanics of the first ray. Part II: metatarsus primus varus as a cause of hypermobility. A three-dimensional kinematic analysis in a cadaver model. J Foot Ankle Surg 2000; 39(Issue 2):68–77.

26. Chan Francis, Bowlby Melinda A, Christensen Jeffrey C. Medial column biomechanics: nonsurgical and surgical implications. Clin Podiatr Med Surg 2020; 37(Issue 1):39–51.

27. Dullaert K, Hagen J, Klos K, et al. The influence of the Peroneus Longus muscle on the foot under axial loading: a CT evaluated dynamic cadaveric model study. Clin Biomech 2016;34:7–11.

28. Johnson Cherie H, Christensen Jeffrey C. Biomechanics of the first ray part V: the effect of equinus deformity: a 3-dimensional kinematic study on a cadaver model. J Foot Ankle Surg 2005;44(Issue 2):114–20.

29. Baxter JR, Demetracopoulos CA, Prado MP, et al. Graft shape affects midfoot correction and forefoot loading mechanics in lateral column lengthening osteotomies. Foot Ankle Int 2014;35(11):1192–9.

30. Deland JT, Page A, Sung IH, et al. Posterior tibial tendon insufficiency results at different stages. HSS Journal® 2006;2(2):157–60.

31. Ellis SJ, Yu JC, Johnson AH, et al. Plantar pressures in patients with and without lateral foot pain after lateral column lengthening. J Bone Joint Surg Am 2010 Jan; 92(1):81–91.

32. Miniaci-Coxhead SL, Weisenthal B, Ketz JP, et al. Incidence and radiographic predictors of valgus tibiotalar tilt after hindfoot fusion. Foot Ankle Int 2017;38(5):519–25.

33. Lin YC, Mhuircheartaigh JN, Lamb J, et al. Imaging of adult flatfoot: correlation of radiographic measurements with MRI. AJR Am J Roentgenol 2015;204(2):354–9.

34. Mackenzie T, Jones BA, Austin E, et al. Assessment of various measurement methods to assess first metatarsal elevation in hallux rigidus. Foot & Ankle Orthopaedics 2019;4. 2473011419875686.

35. Lundgren P, Nester C, Liu A, et al. Invasive in vivo measurement of rear-, mid-and forefoot motion during walking. Gait & posture 2008;28(1):93–100.

36. Joshua A. Metzl,Naviculocuneiform sag in the acquired flatfoot: what to do. Foot Ankle Clin 2017;22(Issue 3):529–44. ISSN 1083-7515,ISBN 9780323545525.

37. Ajis A, Geary N. Surgical technique, fusion rates, and planovalgus foot deformity correction with naviculocuneiform fusion. Foot Ankle Int 2014;35(3):232–7.

38. Astion D.J., Deland J.T., Otis J.C., et al., Motion of the hindfoot after simulated arthrodesis, JBJS, 79 (2), 1997, 241–246.

39. Steiner C.S., Gilgen A., Zwicky L., et al., Combined subtalar and naviculocuneiform fusion for treating adult acquired flatfoot deformity with medial arch collapse at the level of the naviculocuneiform joint, Foot Ankle Int, 40 (1), 2019, 42–47.

40. Southwell RB, Sherman FC. Triple arthrodesis: a long-term study with force plate analysis. Foot & Ankle 1981;2(1):15–24.

41. Scott Ryan T, Bussewitz Bradly W, Hyer Christopher F, et al. The corrective power of the Cotton osteotomy. Fuß & Sprunggelenk 2016;14(Issue 1):9–13.

42. Kunas GC, Do HT, Aiyer A, et al. Contribution of medial cuneiform osteotomy to correction of longitudinal arch collapse in stage iib adult-acquired flatfoot deformity. Foot Ankle Int 2018;39(8):885–93.

43. Kim J-Y, Sic Park J, Hwang SK, et al. Mobility changes of the first ray after hallux valgus surgery: clinical results after proximal metatarsal chevron osteotomy and distal procedure. Foot Ankle Int 2008;29(5):468–72.

44. Cowie S, Parsons S, Scammell B, et al. Hypermobility of the first ray in patients with planovalgus feet and tarsometatarsal osteoarthritis. Foot Ankle Surg 2012; 18:237–40.

45. Johnson T.M., Hentges M.J., McMillen R.L., et al., Effect of the first tarsometatarsal (modified lapidus) arthrodesis on hindfoot alignment, J Foot Ankle Surg, 60 (2), 2021, 318–321.

46. Day J., Conti M.S., Williams N., et al., Contribution of first-tarsometatarsal joint fusion to deformity correction in the treatment of adult-acquired flatfoot deformity, *Foot & Ankle Orthopaedics*, 5 (3), 2020, 2473011420927321.
47. Myerson Mark S, Kadakia Anish R. 14 - correction of flatfoot deformity in the adult, reconstructive foot and ankle surgery: management of complications. 3rd Edition. Elsevier; 2019. p. 194–219.
48. Smits-Engelsman Bouwien, Klerks Mariëtte, Kirby Amanda, et al. A valid measure for generalized hypermobility in children. J Pediatr 2011;158(Issue 1):119–23.e4.
49. Harper MC, Tisdel CL. Talonavicular arthrodesis for the painful adult acquired flatfoot. Foot Ankle Int 1996;17(11):658–61.

Naviculocuneiform Arthrodesis for Treatment of Adult-Acquired Flatfoot Deformity

Jason V. Naldo, DPM[a],*, Kelly Kugach, DPM[b]

KEYWORDS

- Naviculocuneiform arthrodesis • Adult-acquired flatfoot
- Posterior tibial tendon dysfunction • Pes planovalgus • Supinatus

KEY POINTS

- Medial column instability in the adult-acquired flatfoot can involve any combination of the talonavicular, naviculocuneiform, and tarsometatarsal joints.
- Proper evaluation of the medial column preoperatively can be difficult when multiple joints of the medial column are involved.
- Fusion of the naviculocuneiform joint, either in concert with other medial column joints or in isolation, is a reliable option for stabilization of the medial column.

INTRODUCTION

Adult-acquired flat foot (AAFF) is a complex multiplanar deformity that involves rearfoot valgus, forefoot varus, forefoot abduction, and medial column collapse. AAFF has many etiologies including arthritis, trauma, and the most common cause being posterior tibial tendon dysfunction.[1] On the basis of the chronicity of the pathology, as well as the severity of deformity, multiple joints can be involved in the structural malalignment of the AAFF. As rearfoot protonation and hindfoot valgus worsen over time, the forefoot will supinate to maintain purchase with the ground, ultimately resulting in medial column instability. This instability of the medial longitudinal arch can involve the talonavicular (TN), naviculocuneiform (NC), or tarsometatarsal (TMT) joints to varying degrees. When surgical reconstruction of the AAFF is necessary, arthrodesis of the NC joint, either isolated or incorporated into a medial column

[a] Department of Orthopaedics, Virginia Tech Carilion, School of Medicine, Carilion Clinic Institute for Orthopaedics & Neurosciences, 2900 Lamb Circle, Suite L-760, Christiansburg, VA 24073, USA; [b] Carilion Clinic, Institute for Orthopaedics & Neurosciences, 1906 Belleview Avenue, Med Ed 202, Roanoke, VA 24014, USA
* Corresponding author.
E-mail address: jvnaldo@carilionclinic.org

Clin Podiatr Med Surg 40 (2023) 293–305
https://doi.org/10.1016/j.cpm.2022.11.004
0891-8422/23/© 2022 Elsevier Inc. All rights reserved.

arthrodesis, has shown to be a reliable and reproducible option for the foot and ankle surgeon[2–6]

FUNCTIONAL ANATOMY OF THE NAVICULOCUNEIFORM JOINT

The NC joint is composed of the distal aspect of the navicular articulating with three cuneiforms, each with individual facets. The navicular is pyriform in shape, with the long axis oblique in nature, directed downward and medially. The anterior surface of the navicular is entirely articular with the cuneiforms and is angular and faceted, yet convex in its general contour. Each cuneiform is wedge-shaped with its base located dorsally and the apex plantar.[7–9] The NC joint is reinforced by both dorsal and plantar ligamentous attachments. All three NC joints are held within one joint capsule.

Hansen has labeled the NC joint as not only nonessential but unnecessary for normal gait, indicating that loss of motion in the NC joint would have no significant effect on a patient's normal gait.[10] There is evidence that the range of motion obtained through the NC joint is likely underappreciated, bringing into question the theory of the joint being nonessential. Multiple studies have evaluated a sagittal plane range of motion of the medial column, and it has been found that the NC joint not only provides 50% of the total sagittal plane range of motion, but the NC joint also shows a 12.2° of sagittal plane range of motion, which is significantly more than both the TN and TMT joints.[11,12] As noted, the primary plane of motion of the NC joint is the sagittal plane, although some frontal plane range of motion does occur as it was found on weight-bearing CT analysis that the medial cuneiform pronates 6.1° relative to the navicular at the NC joint. The medial cuneiform rotates in the frontal plane significantly less than the other bones in the medial column, as the navicular and proximal first metatarsal each rotate at 43.2° and 33.9°, respectively.[13] Although a large proportion of the medial column range of motion is obtained through the NC joint, it has also been shown that stabilization of the NC joint has no effect on TN or TMT joint range of motion, essentially confirming Hansen's determination that the NC is unnecessary for normal gait.[11]

NAVICULOCUNEIFORM JOINT'S ROLE IN FLATFOOT DEFORMITY

The biomechanics and pathophysiology of medial column collapse have been well established in the literature, as rearfoot protonation leads to unlocking of the oblique axis of the midtarsal joint. This unstable midtarsal joint then compensates for the rearfoot protonation by supinating the forefoot along the long axis of the midtarsal joint for the forefoot to maintain ground purchase.[2] As this process becomes chronic in nature, acquired soft tissue contracture occurs leading to forefoot supinatus deformity, whereby the long-standing soft tissue adaptation creates a supinated forefoot. This becomes a more rigid forefoot varus deformity over an extended period of time as the soft tissue adaptive changes lead to degenerative changes in the articular surfaces of the medial column joints.[2] These changes can vary regarding which joints are involved, and the key to proper surgical decision-making is to ensure that the surgical plan includes correcting the joints that lead to the deformity.

NAVICULOCUNEIFORM ARTHRODESIS FOR THE TREATMENT OF FLATFOOT DEFORMITY

In the literature today, NC arthrodesis has been shown to help recreate and stabilize the medial arch as well as improve Meary's angle.[3,4,14] It is of utmost importance for the foot and ankle surgeon to ensure that if surgical reconstruction of the AAFF is to be undertaken, the procedure that is chosen correct the joints that are involved in the patient's specific deformity. There is no single protocol that all patients will fit in to when making decisions regarding surgical planning for the AAFF. Age, body habitus, postoperative activity goals, medical comorbidities, as well as clinical and radiographic evaluation all play a vital role in the decision-making process.

CLINICAL EVALUATION

Physicians should thoroughly evaluate patients with adult-acquired flatfoot to determine the biomechanical etiology of the deformity. It is important to evaluate patients in weight-bearing and non-weight-bearing scenarios.

For the non-weight-bearing examination, assessment of the ankle range of motion for presence of equinus is an important diagnostic step to determine if lengthening of the gastroc-soleal construct is necessary. One must also evaluate for spasm or contracture of the peroneal tendons, as spasm may indicate presence of a tarsal coalition and contracture may warrant lengthening or peroneal tendon transfer. The further non-weight-bearing examination includes palpation along the posterior tibial tendon, assessing for pain and hypertrophy of the tendon, as well as manipulation of the midtarsal, NC, and TMT joints. To assess for forefoot supination, the surgeon should hold the subtalar joint in the neutral position and evaluate the relative position of the first ray (**Fig. 1**). Significant forefoot varus indicates the presence of forefoot supinatus. Although somewhat controversial, hypermobility of the medial column should also be assessed. It has been suggested that if you can elevate the first metatarsal head greater than 10 mm above the second metatarsal head, the medial column should be considered hypermobile[15] (**Fig. 2**). Crepitus upon manipulation of the subtalar, midtarsal, NC, and TMT joints also indicates degenerative changes, which is important in surgical planning.

Weight-bearing examination includes viewing the patient in a relaxed stance both posteriorly and superiorly. Posterior/axial evaluation can reveal valgus position of the heel as well as midfoot abduction via the "too many toes" sign[16] (**Fig. 3**). The patient should then be asked to perform a heel rise to determine flexibility of the heel valgus, as well as the strength of the Achilles and posterior tibial tendons. In the flexible deformity, the heel will return to neutral upon heel rise (**Fig. 4**). Anterior/superior evaluation can assess for abduction through the midfoot as well as position of the medial longitudinal arch (**Fig. 5**).

RADIOGRAPHIC EVALUATION

Radiographic evaluation of the NC joint includes standard weight-bearing x-rays including AP, lateral, medial oblique. The importance of weight-bearing cannot be understated, especially for the lateral view to determine deformity and instability through the medial column. Traditionally, Meary's angle has been used to evaluate apex of the medial column deformity by assessing the relationship between the long axis of the talus to the long axis of the first metatarsal (**Fig. 6**). A negative Mary's angle of 5°or more indicates significant loss of medial column alignment.[1] However, if multiple joints are involved to find the apex of the deformity, it can be difficult using this method of assessment Another technique that should be employed is to evaluate the long axis of the talus and the long axis of the first metatarsal relative to the body of the navicular (**Fig. 7**). If the long axis of the talus exits the TN joint through the inferior half of the navicular body, there is a significant sagittal plane deformity at the TN joint, with the navicular dorsally displaced on the talar head. If the long axis of the first metatarsal, through the center of the proximal articular surface, exits the navicular cuneiform joint

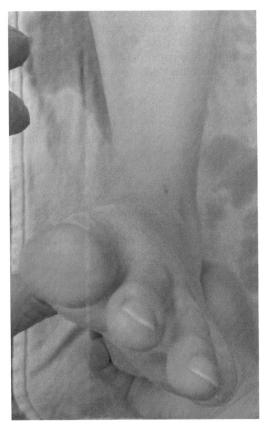

Fig. 1. Reducing the heel valgus and correcting midfoot abduction in the open chain evaluation reveals significant forefoot supination.

through the superior portion of the navicular body, then the navicular cuneiform joint is involved with dorsal displacement of the cuneiform on the navicular.[15] This method can be helpful to determine if multiple joints are involved and which joints should be incorporated into reconstruction. Further evaluation of arthritic changes at the navicular cuneiform joints can be noted on both the AP and lateral views with dorsal exostosis and subchondral sclerosis (**Figs. 8** and **9**). Significant plantar gapping of the first TMT joint may also indicate a need for arthrodesis of the joint secondary to instability (**Fig. 10**).

Advanced imaging can give further insight into the involvement of the arthritic component to the NC joint. Specifically, computed tomography (CT) should be used when there is concern regarding significant degenerative changes and if those joints need to be incorporated into reconstruction. Common findings on the CT scan will be subchondral cysts, asymmetric joint space wearing, and dorsal exostosis at the NC joint. This author does not find significant value in MRI for this specific pathology.

OPERATIVE CONSIDERATIONS

Once it has been determined that the NC joint should be part of the reconstructive plan, there are some important decision-making points the surgeon must consider. Whether the NC will couple with TN or TMT arthrodesis, the surgeon must decide if

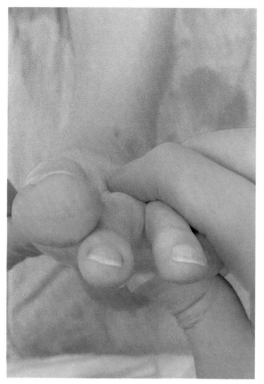

Fig. 2. Hypermobility of the medial column shown by elevation of the first metatarsal head relative to the second metatarsal head.

fusion of the medial cuneiform-navcular (MCN) articulation alone or if the intermediate (ICN) and lateral cuneiform (LCN) articulations should be included. There is no evidence supporting one technique over the other, and surgeon preference and experience will play a role in this decision; however, the techniques are vastly different. If the MCN articulation is to be fused without the involvement of the intermediate or lateral

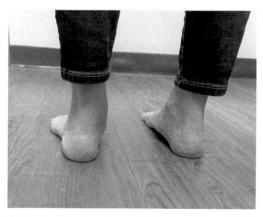

Fig. 3. Posterior/axial visualization showing medial arch collapse, hindfoot valgus, and positive "too many toes sign" of the left foot.

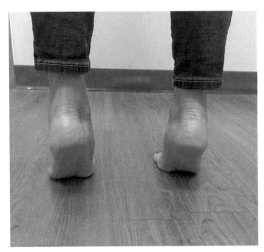

Fig. 4. Bipedal heel rise showing inversion of the subtalar joint, confirming a flexible deformity.

cuneiform joints, the surgeon should be aware that primary fusion without use of bone graft will not be possible, as the intercuneiform articulation will not allow proximal migration of the medial cuneiform. Of note, it has been shown that fusion of the medial–intermediate cuneiform joint decreases rotation of the first ray significantly, providing a more stable medial column.[11]

SURGICAL TECHNIQUE
Incision Placement

Incision placement will vary depending on if the NC joint will be an isolated procedure or incorporated in a multi-joint medial column arthrodesis. For the isolated arthrodesis, an incision placed at the dorsal/medial midfoot, directly superior to the medial cuneiform and between the tibialis anterior and extensor hallucis longus tendon, provides the best exposure to all three joints (**Fig. 11**). Placing the incision too medial can create

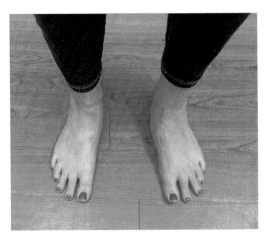

Fig. 5. Anterior/superior visualization showing collapse of the medial arch and abduction through the midfoot of the left foot.

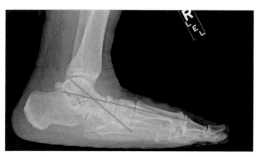

Fig. 6. Lateral projection of patient with AAFF assessing traditional Meary's angle, indicating an apex of deformity in the talus (Lateral Talo-First Metatarsal Angle).

difficulty with visualization of the LCN articulation. This approach allows for clear visualization of the NC joint without concern for damage to any major neurovascular structure. When performing a multi-joint medial column fusion, a medial utility incision, from the talar nick to the mid-diaphyseal region of the first metatarsal is appropriate. Although this is less than ideal for access to the lateral potion of the NC joint, the incision is typically long enough to develop a full-thickness soft tissue window dorsally to allow visualization. Use of appropriate joint distractors improves visualization as well when the incision is placed medially.

Joint Preparation

Standard techniques for joint preparation including curettage, ronguer, osteotomes, and power burr can be used as per surgeon preference. It should be noted that if plantarflexion osteotomy through the joint is to be performed that a sagittal saw can also be used but care must be taken to avoid too much shortening through the joint. If a complete NC joint fusion is being performed, preparation of the intercuneiform joints is not necessary (**Fig. 12**).

Definitive Stabilization

As with any arthrodesis procedure, definitive fixation devices are chosen based on surgeon comfort and experience. Screws, locking plates, and staples are all viable

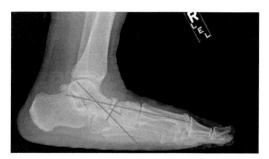

Fig. 7. Lateral projection of patient (same patient as **Fig. 7**) with AAFF assessing relative axis of the talus and first metatarsal to the bisection of the navicular body. The axis of the talus falls below the bisection of the navicular body revealing dorsal subluxation of the talonavicular joint. The axis of the first metatarsal falls above the bisection of the navicular body revealing dorsal subluxation of the NC joint. This indicates multiple joint involvement and the lack of a single "apex" of deformity.

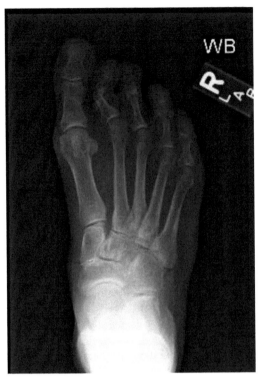

Fig. 8. AP projection of patient with AAFF revealing degenerative changes at the NC and intercuneiform joints.

options; however, there is evidence that some constructs are more stable than others. It has been shown that for each NC joint, use of crossed lag screws or a combination of one lag screw and a locking plate both significantly decrease rotation of joint being fused, without effect of rotation for the adjacent joints.[17] Furthermore, incorporation of an intercuneiform screw has also been noted to decrease rotation throughout the whole medial column.[11] The use of nickel-titanium-alloy staples has also increased in the foot and ankle, and these constructs have been noted to provide more contact force and a greater contact area across the arthrodesis site when compared with crossed screws or compress plates.[18] Plantar plating has also been described for the NC joint with good short-term results noted[5] (**Fig. 13**).

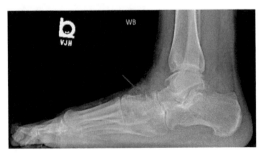

Fig. 9. Lateral projection of patient with AAFF revealing degenerative changes at the NC joint. Degenerative joint changes at the naviculocunieform joint.

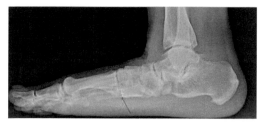

Fig. 10. Lateral projection of patient with AAFF revealing subtle plantar gaping at the first TMT joint. Degenerative joint changes at the naviculocunieform joint.

Postoperative Protocol

Patients are typically immobilized in a well-padded posterior splint with the foot at neutral to the ankle for the initial 2 weeks postoperatively. Transition to a short leg cast occurs after the sutures are removed at 2 weeks and the patient remains non-weight-bearing for a total of 8 weeks. Once the patient is weight-bearing and comfortable, physical therapy is initiated for strengthening, gait, balance, and proprioception training. It is important that the patient understands that the process of rehabilitation back to "normal" can take up to 1 year postoperatively. It is important to emphasize that not only do we have to rehabilitate the newly reconstructed foot, but that there

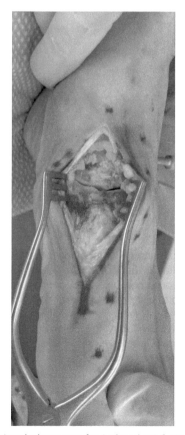

Fig. 11. Dorsal/medial incisional placement for isolated NC fusion.

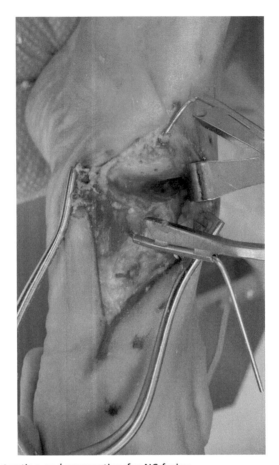

Fig. 12. Joint distraction and preparation for NC fusion.

is significant muscle atrophy of the whole lower extremity while the patient is non-weight-bearing for the immediate postoperative phase, and a full return to preoperative levels of strength will take time.

Complications

The same general complications to all foot and ankle surgery apply to NC fusion. These include wound healing issues, hardware failure, malunion, and nonunion. Of these potential complications, non-union appears to be the most prevalent. NC arthrodesis has been noted to have a nonunion rate of 6.5%.[19] Luckily, with correction of midfoot deformity, the soft tissue along the medial aspect of the midfoot is typically decompressed, leading to a more forgiving incision and minimal risk of incisional complications. The surgeon should take care to maintain the insertion of the tibial anterior tendon to the medial cuneiform to avoid biomechanical imbalance in dorsiflexion and inversion postoperatively.

DISCUSSION

Surgical reconstruction of the adult flat foot deformity is complex, and procedure choice is of the utmost importance for the foot & ankle surgeon. Along with structural

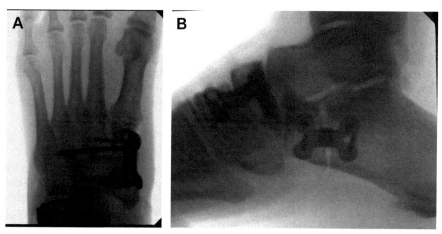

Fig. 13. Definitive stabilization of isolated NC fusion. (A) AP view of NC fusion stabilized with medial compression plate. (B) Lateral view of NC fusion coupled with Evans calcaneal osteotomy.

realignment, tendon balancing procedures are also necessary to allow proper mechanics postoperatively. Achilles tendon lengthening alone has been shown to significantly improve calcaneal inclination angle and Meary's angle.[20] Transfer of the peroneus brevis tendon to decrease eversion force has also started to gain traction among foot and ankle surgeons.[21] Although arthrodesis of the NC joint is a powerful

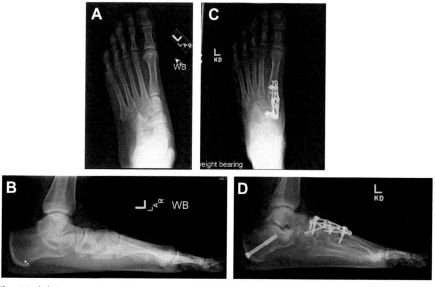

Fig. 14. (A) Preoperative AP projection of patient with AAFF and significant medial column instability. (B) Preoperative lateral projection of patient with AAFF and significant medial column instability. (C) Postoperative AP projection following AAFF reconstruction with double calcaneal osteotomy (Evans & Medial Displacement Calcaneal Osteotomy) and medial column fusion including NC and TMT joints. (D) Postoperative lateral projection following AAFF reconstruction with double calcaneal osteotomy (Evans & Medial Displacement Calcaneal Osteotomy) and medial column fusion including NC and TMT joints.

procedure to realign and stabilize the medial column, it is rarely used as an isolated procedure alone. Along with the soft tissue balancing procedures alone, NC arthrodesis combined with lateral column lengthening, subtalar fusion, and concomitant medial column arthrodesis have yielded reliable results (**Fig. 14**).[4,13,14] It is key that the surgeon corrects the underlying biomechanical factors that contribute to NC instability. Without correction of heel valgus, hypermobility of the subtalar joint, and ankle equinus, the NC fusion will ultimately fail to provide the patient with long-term stability of the medial longitudinal arch.

SUMMARY

Arthrodesis of the NC joint is a powerful tool for the foot & ankle surgeon during the reconstruction of the adult-acquired flatfoot. Medial column instability, forefoot supination, and degenerative changes at the NC joint are all indications for incorporating the NC fusion into the surgical plan. Proper clinical and radiographic evaluation is imperative to ensure that the appropriate procedures are performed during reconstruction. The surgical techniques have been described and results of NC fusion are reliable and successful in improving pain, quality of life, and function for patients.

CLINICS CARE POINTS

- Naviculocuneiform (NC) arthrodesis is an often overlooked option for stabilizing the medial column
- The unique shape of the articular surfaces of the NC joints can create difficult with full exposure without proper incision placement
- Stabilization of the NC fusion can be achieved with isolated NC joint fixation or with constructs that span multiple joints and/or the medial column
- Neglecting to include NC arthrodesis in patients where arthritis or joint instability is present increases the risk of recurrence of medial column collapse.

DISCLOSURE

The authors have no financial disclosures relative to this article.

REFERENCES

1. McCormick JJ, Johnson JE. Medial column procedures in the correction of adult acquired flatfoot deformity. Foot Ankle Clin 2012;17(2):283–98.
2. Evans EL, Catanzariti AR. Forefoot supinatus. Clin Podiatr Med Surg 2014;31(3): 405–13.
3. Gerrity M, Williams M. Naviculocuneiform arthrodesis in adult flatfoot: a case series. J Foot Ankle Surg 2019;58(2):352–6.
4. Steiner CS, Gilgen A, Zwicky L, et al. Combined subtalar and naviculocuneiform fusion for treating adult acquired flatfoot deformity with medial arch collapse at the level of the naviculocuneiform joint. Foot Ankle Int 2019;40(1):42–7.
5. Wininger AE, Klavas DM, Gardner SS, et al. Plantar plating for medial naviculocuneiform arthrodesis in progressive collapsing foot deformity. Foot Ankle Orthop 2022;7(1). 24730114221088517.
6. Cohen BE, Ogden F. Medial column procedures in the acquired flatfoot deformity. Foot Ankle Clin 2007;12(2):287–99.

7. Kelikian AS, Sarrafian SK, Sarrafian SK. Sarrafian's anatomy of the foot and ankle: descriptive, topographical, functional. Philadelphia: Wolters Kluwer Health/Lippincott Williams & Wilkins; 2011. Print.

8. Casciato D, Yancovitz S, Olivová J, et al. Anatomic description of the distal and intercuneiform articulations: a cadaveric study. J Foot Ankle Surg 2021;60(6): 1137–43.

9. Borrelli GJ, Qatu M, Traynor CJ, et al. Anatomy of the naviculocuneiform joint. Foot Ankle Orthop 2022;7(1). 2473011421S00119.

10. Hansen ST. Functional reconstruction of the foot and ankle. Philadelphis: Lippincott Williams & Wilkins; 2000.

11. Roling BA, Christensen JC, Johnson CH. Biomechanics of the first ray. Part IV: the effect of selected medial column arthrodeses. A three-dimensional kinematic analysis in a cadaver model. J Foot Ankle Surg 2002;41(5):278–85.

12. Whittaker EC, Aubin PM, Ledoux WR. Foot bone kinematics as measured in a cadaveric robotic gait simulator. Gait Posture 2011;33(4):645–50.

13. Schmidt E, Silva T, Baumfeld D, et al. The rotational positioning of the bones in the medial column of the foot: a weightbearing CT analysis. Iowa Orthop J 2021; 41(1):103–9.

14. Ajis A, Geary N. Surgical technique, fusion rates, and planovalgus foot deformity correction with naviculocuneiform fusion. Foot Ankle Int 2014;35(3):232–7.

15. Boberg JS, McMurray SJ. Evaluation of the medial column in flatfoot surgery. Clin Podiatr Med Surg 2007;24(4):721–33.

16. Sanhudo JAV. Dynamic correction for forefoot varus in stage II-A adult flatfoot: technique tip. Foot Ankle Surg 2019;25(5):698–700.

17. Kuestermann H, Ettinger S, Yao D, et al. Biomechanical evaluation of naviculocuneiform fixation with lag screw and locking plates. Foot Ankle Surg 2021;27(8): 911–9.

18. Aiyer A, Russell NA, Pelletier MH, et al. The impact of nitinol staples on the compressive forces, contact area, and mechanical properties in comparison to a claw plate and crossed screws for the first tarsometatarsal arthrodesis. Foot Ankle Spec 2016;9(3):232–40.

19. Chu AK, Wilson MD, Lee J, et al. The incidence of nonunion of the naviculocuneiform joint arthrodesis: A systematic review. J Foot Ankle Surg 2019;58(3):545–9.

20. Kim NT, Lee YT, Park MS, et al. Changes in the bony alignment of the foot after tendo-Achilles lengthening in patients with planovalgus deformity. J Orthop Surg Res 2021;16(1):118.

21. Budny AM, Grossman JP. Naviculocuneiform arthrodesis. Clin Podiatr Med Surg 2007;24(4):753–63.

Ligament Insufficiency with Flatfoot

Spring Ligament and Deltoid Ligament

Sara Mateen, DPM, AACFAS[a], Jennifer C. Van, DPM, MBA, FACFAS[b],*

KEYWORDS

- Deltoid ligament • Spring ligament • Flatfoot deformity • Ligament insufficiency
- Foot surgery • Ankle surgery • Talocalcaneonavicular • Ligamentous repair

KEY POINTS

- Recognize the normal biomechanical forces extending through the deltoid and spring ligament during their physiologic function.
- Understand the spring ligament complex and the deltoid ligament as it pertains to medial column stability.
- Appreciate the literature in terms of surgical augmentation and repair of the medial ligamentous structures for flatfoot reconstruction.

INTRODUCTION

Adult-acquired flatfoot deformity (AAFD) is a common clinical condition that can present with mild-to-severe functional limitations with subsequent development of arthritis.[1,2] Approximately 1% of the population with AAFD are symptomatic with a peak age of around 55 years old.[3–7] A thorough history is important as patients will often report pain along the medial arch and under/inside the ankle and as symptoms progress, patients will note their arch has fallen in conjunction with pain along the lateral ankle. Patients may also describe increased pain with activity and pain with certain shoe wear. In mild symptomatic patients, conservative treatment such as orthotics or non-custom braces may be beneficial.[3–7] As the symptoms progress, however, patients may require surgical intervention for optimal return to function.[8]

When assessing the patient, the Johnson and Strom, Bluman, and Myerson classifications are useful in guiding surgical intervention with an appropriate mix of osseous and soft tissue procedures.[9,10] Posterior tibial tendon dysfunction (PTTD) begins with stage I, which involves mild to moderate pain along the course of the posterior tibial

a Foot and Ankle Deformity and Orthoplastics, Rubin Institute for Advanced Orthopedics, Baltimore, MD, USA; b Department of Podiatric Surgery, Temple University School of Podiatric Medicine, 148 North 8th Street, Philadelphia, PA 19107, USA
* Corresponding author.
E-mail address: jvan@temple.edu

Clin Podiatr Med Surg 40 (2023) 307–314
https://doi.org/10.1016/j.cpm.2022.11.008
podiatric.theclinics.com

(PT) tendon with normal hindfoot alignment. Radiographs are typically normal, but an MRI may show inflammation of the PT tendon. Stage II progresses into a more flexible flatfoot deformity with the loss of the ability to perform a single heel raise.[9,10] The medial arch begins to collapse secondary to the failure of the spring ligament and the PT tendon. Owing to the PT tendon weakness, the transverse tarsal joints are unable to lock and engage for heel raise and eventually, forefoot abduction, hindfoot valgus, and forefoot varus may occur. Stage III flatfoot is a rigid deformity of the subtalar, talonavicular, and calcaneocuboid joints that will not correct with a passive range of motion with concurrent radiographic changes consistent with arthritis.[9,10] The forefoot is fixed in abduction and patients will have fixed hindfoot valgus with subfibular impingement. Finally, stage IV flatfoot deformity is seen with tibiotalar valgus with asymmetric tibiotalar arthritis with similar features of stage III.[9,10]

The objective of this review was to provide a critical assessment of the literature with respect to the tibiocalcaneonavicular ligament and deltoid ligament complex as they pertain to AAFD, specifically in flexible deformity. Tibiocalcaneonavicular ligament (spring ligament) tears are common in AAFD. Recent studies suggest that the spring ligament may play a role in peritalar medial stability. Given its essential role in providing medial tibiotalar and talonavicular stability in advanced AAFD, these ligaments may collectively become attenuated and lead to instability. This review also critically assesses the literature as it pertains to spring ligament and deltoid ligament repair in flatfoot deformity reconstructive surgery.

THE SPRING LIGAMENT

The spring ligament complex (SLC) is a thick triangular anatomic structure that connects to the sustentaculum tali of the calcaneus to the navicular.[11-15] There are two distinct ligamentous bands of the spring ligament: the superomedial calcaneonavicular (SMCN) ligament is a fibrocartilaginous band with collagen orientation to withstand repetitive loads, whereas the inferomedial calcaneonavicular (IMCN) ligament presents organized longitudinal fibers to resist tensile forces are the major portions of the SLC.[12] The plantar portion of the PT tendon provides some support to the inferior spring ligament and laterally, it is contiguous with the medial band of the bifurcate ligament. The main function of the SLC involves supporting the head of the talus, providing static stability to the talar head and the talonavicular joint, supporting the medial longitudinal arch, and providing kinetic coupling between the forefoot and the hindfoot.[16-18] There is an intimate relationship with the tibiospring ligament from the deltoid complex that further contributes to the full SLC. This highlights the importance of repairing the deltoid complex in SLC compromise.[14,16-23]

AAFD was traditionally thought to occur secondary to PTTD; however, recent studies have stressed the importance of static stability as shown by the spring ligament.[2-4,24-30] PTTD can lead to an increased stress over the medial structures of the foot and ankle, which can eventually progress to the failure of the SLC and the development of talonavicular deformity.[24-30] Tears or attenuation of the SLC, most commonly the SMCN ligament, is found in approximately 70% with some deformity secondary to PTTD.[24-31] Tryfonidis and colleagues saw SLC insufficiency in patients who performed a single heel raise appropriately with partial restoration of the medial arch. These patients, however, had persistent forefoot abduction and heel valgus with more anterior medial malleolar pain versus the typical posterior-inferior tenderness found along the PT tendon.[32]

Other indications for spring ligament compromise include medial foot pain which can be caused secondary to trauma. The neutral heel test has been described by Pasapula and colleagues[16] to determine the SLC integrity. Twenty-one cadavers were assessed for lateral translation of the midfoot when applying a lateral force to the medial midfoot with graduated anterograde and retrograde de-functioning of the PT tendon and the flexor digitorum longus (FDL) tendon while keeping the tibiotalar joint in dorsiflexion and second toe aligned to the tibial shaft or in slight varus.[16] Based on cadaveric results, greater lateral translation occurred in all specimens when the SLC was incised. Overall, the study showed the SLC was the primary supporting structure, and an isolated PT tendon rupture would not lead to lateral translation without de-functioning the SLC.[16] The midfoot is the main connection of the two longitudinal arches after they bifurcate at the heel before they re-diverge from each other the five metatarsals, thus playing a vital role in the loading change between these two segments.[3,4,33]

The anatomic position of the midfoot along with the spring ligament is equally important to biomechanics of gait.[29] This is particularly true with the navicular. Cifuentes-De la Portilla and colleagues[29] used a finite-element model to evaluate different flatfoot arthrodesis treatments and visualize the different stresses on the bone and cartilage in relation to each procedure. According to their findings, the increased stress of the navicular was largely due to the spring ligament. This illustrates the importance of the SLC on overall foot structure and shows that the tensile strength of cancellous bone was only 70% of compressive strength.[29] The results of the study also suggest that injury or rupture of the spring ligament could increase the plantar arch fall by about 14.9%, concluding that the spring ligament is the second most important tissue in the plantar maintenance. Cheung and colleagues[34] showed that force loaded on the spring ligament was approximately 50N during two-foot balance and gait; while with single-foot stance, the force increased to 82N. This validates the biomechanical importance of an intact spring ligament for repair.[34]

THE DELTOID LIGAMENT

The deltoid ligament is the primary stabilizer of the ankle joint, and the spring ligament is the main static supporter of the medial longitudinal arch. Therefore, many publications have supported correcting both of these ligaments for appropriate treatment.[3,4] Deland and colleagues[31] reviewed MRI imaging with flatfoot deformity and found that PT tendon dysfunction was pathologic in 100% of patients, the superomedial components of the spring ligament in 87%, inferior spring ligament in 74%, talocalcaneal interosseous in 48%, anterior superficial deltoid, the deep deltoid, and the posterior superficial deltoid in 33%. Malakoutikhah and colleagues[22] evaluated the contributions of each ligament in the maintenance of foot alignment using computed tomography scan images Based on their results, the plantar fascia, deltoid, and spring ligaments were primarily responsible for preventing medial arch collapse, hindfoot valgus, and forefoot abduction and that single ligament failure of one of these ligaments may not contribute enough to the development of AAFD.[22]

Nery and colleagues described the correction of AAFD with the combination of deltoid and spring ligament repair using bone anchors and fibertape suture in the medial malleolus, sustentaculum tali, and the talar neck.[21] All patients had clinical improvement of their pain level and return to normal activity with a mean AOFAS score from 23 preoperatively to 86 postoperatively (Neary). The talar first metatarsal angle, talonavicular uncovering, talar pitch, calcaneal pitch, talonavicular sag on the lateral view all significantly improved postoperatively.[21] Similarly, to the Neary study, Lui and colleagues described an endoscopic repair with the proximal and distal portals along the tendon sheath with the proximal portal located 1 cm proximal to the medial malleolar tip and the distal portal located close to the navicular insertion of the tendon.[20,26] Although this technique can repair both the deltoid and spring ligaments along with repair of the PT tendon, this surgical system can be technically challenging to perform.[20,26] Deltoid ligament repair can also aid in ankle joint preservation in the setting of a triple arthrodesis. Oburo and Myerson[27] discussed in their publication that although there are increased forces that may occur across the ankle joint after a triple arthrodesis, deltoid ligament reconstruction may delay or even present the onset of arthritis. The authors also noted that deltoid ligament repair may also allow the patient to maintain mobility of the ankle joint after hindfoot fusion, again recognizing the importance of deltoid ligament repair in AAFD.[27]

AAFD can be treated in several ways but mainly depends on the clinical and radiographic findings[24–30] It is important to categorize these deformities in stages as shown by the Johnson and Strom classification. Repair of the SLC is usually reported as an adjunctive procedure for stage IIB flatfoot deformity along with other conventional procedures such as the medial calcaneal slide osteotomy, lateral column lengthening osteotomy, and FDL tendon transfer. These procedures have their individual indications for overall reconstruction; however, these procedures do not reconstitute the plantar arch as effectively as primarily SLC repair. The concept of supraphysiologic construct is important as it pertains to superior surgical repairs to aid in quicker return to function and patient satisfaction. Secondary procedures are needed if osseous correction is indicated, but recent literature has expressed interest in direct SLC repair for optimal biomechanical correction.[35–38]

The question of whether perform the direct repair of the spring ligament or repair with augmentation also raises the point of which one would provide supraphysiologic repair. Several studies have been discussed for direct repair versus augmentation of the spring ligament. Pasapula and colleagues compared a simple spring ligament repair as well as an augmented spring ligament repair with the FDL tendon.[16] Their findings showed little added biomechanical strength to the repair construct and the addition of an internal brace device also adds resistance to lateral translation.[16] The combined anatomic repair of the spring ligament and the deltoid augmentation with the FDL transfer is also of importance because the SLC involves the deltoid ligament and helps function as a biomechanical unit versus a euphysiologic simple repair of the deltoid ligament. Other publications have also been in support of spring ligament augmentation and repair. Deland and colleagues described a deltoid ligament block bone graft from the medial malleolus that preserved the insertion of the superficial portion of the deltoid ligament on the sustentaculum tali. The bone block then attaches to the navicular and with manipulation, the authors concluded that this procedure aids in maintaining good correction.[31] Choi and colleagues[35] used the peroneus longus tendon to recreate the SLC and then combined superomedial/plantar passage of the tendon through the calcaneus and the navicular. The authors concluded that this method was more effective and helped correct the talonavicular joint to adducted position. Ellis and colleagues similarly looked at 13 patients (14 feet) undergoing flatfoot surgery and they used the peroneus tendon transfer as an augmentation to spring ligament repair in cases where the lateral column lengthening osteotomy failed to correct forefoot abduction.[36]

When analyzing the biomechanical forces of each isolated joint after arthrodesis, Cifuentes-De la Portilla and colleagues found that the talonavicular joint fusion generated a significant stress reduction as compared with the subtalar joint fusion that would offer the least amount of stress reduction. Again, to the point of anatomic locations of fixation, the spring ligament and deltoid (tibiotalar) ligament complex is important to fixation primarily with augmentation for increased biomechanical stability.[30] Another supporting publication performed by Aynardi and colleagues who used fibertape for spring ligament augmentation.[25] The authors found that under cyclic loading and ground reaction force magnitudes under 1,600N provided no significant differences between the traditional spring ligament augmentation and fibertape, which again, supports direct repair of this ligament.[25]

SURGICAL CONSIDERATIONS

When critically analyzing the literature, one might argue that direct spring ligament repair with augmentation may provide supraphysiologic repair as the primary supporting structure of the medial longitudinal arch and the talonavicular joint. A combined spring and deltoid ligament repair was first described by Grunfeld and colleagues in which the authors noted that medial column peritalar instability should be addressed with AAFD in combination with other procedures for maximum repair.[37] In addition to the spring ligament playing a role in peritalar stability, the tibiocalcaneonavicular ligament aids in stability of the tibiotalar, talonavicular, and subtalar joints. Raikin and Rogero compared patients with direct repair of a spring ligament versus those with a tear without repair.[38] Based on their results, the authors concluded that increased patient age, increased talo-navicular coverage, and decreasing talonavicular angle are independent associated with increased likelihood of having AAFD with a spring ligament tear.[38] It should also be noted that the authors did not find a clinically significant difference between those spring ligament tears repaired and those without repair.[38]

Growing evidence in the literature suggests that spring ligament reconstruction can provide excellent clinical and radiographic correction with re-establishment of the ligamentous structures of the medial arch.[14] Brodell and colleagues looked at two different spring ligament reconstruction techniques with tendon allograft and found that there was improved peritalar stability with improved radiographic and patient-reported outcomes at 2 years' follow-up.[39] Fogelman and colleagues hypothesized that suture tape augmentation will strengthen the spring ligament repair and to their results, found an improved talocalcaneal angle, talo-first metatarsal angle, talonavicular coverage, medial cuneiform-first metatarsal height, and calcaneal pitch.[40] Similarly, to Brodell and Fogelman, Tang and Ng compared patients that underwent spring ligament suture tape augmentation with an FDL transfer to those with an FDL transfer alone or with a medial calcaneal osteotomy.[41] Compared with the control groups, the suture tape augmentation group had excellent patient functional outcomes as well as postoperative radiographic parameters.[41]

As previously noted, both the spring ligament and superficial deltoid ligament work together to stabilize the medial ankle and foot. A compromised SLC is a causative factor of talar de-rotation that leads to peritalar subluxation. A few publications have discussed the repair of both the spring ligament and the deltoid ligament for excellent postoperative outcomes of flatfoot reconstruction.[21,42–44] Nery and colleagues described a "novel" technique to reconstruct the deltoid and spring ligament at the same time using suture tape augmentation. Based on their results, there were no postoperative complications, stiffness, or loss of correction.[21] Similarly, Acevedo and Vora used an "internal brace" suture tape augmentation of the SLC with good postoperative clinical results.[43] Macdonald and colleagues assessed the biomechanical effect of the spring ligament on peritalar stability as well as the effect of the talocalcaneonavicular complex (TCNL) ligament reconstruction with medial stabilization of the deltoid ligament. Based on their cadaveric results, the TCNL complex provided stability to the talonavicular, subtalar, and tibiotalar joints and the combined deltoid-spring ligament reconstruction restored the peritalar kinematics better than isolated spring ligament or deltoid ligament in severe AAFD.[44]

SUMMARY

Tibiocalcaneonavicular ligament (spring ligament) tears are common in AAFD. Recent studies suggest that the spring ligament may play a role in peritalar medial stability and given its essential role in providing medial tibiotalar and talonavicular stability in advanced AAFD, these ligaments may collectively become attenuated and lead to instability. Both the spring ligament and superficial deltoid ligament work together to stabilize the medial ankle and foot. Surgical repair of both the spring ligament and the deltoid ligament is important for excellent postoperative outcomes in flatfoot reconstruction.

CLINICS CARE POINTS

- Spring and deltoid ligaments play a role in peritalar medial stability and given its essential role in providing medial tibiotalar and talonavicular stability in advanced AAFD.
- Surgical repair of both the spring ligament and the deltoid ligament is important for excellent postoperative outcomes in flatfoot reconstruction.

DISCLOSURE

All authors have no financial disclosures to report.

REFERENCES

1. Henry JK, Shakked R, Ellis SJ. Adult-acquired flatfoot deformity. Foot Ankle Orthop 2019;4(1). 2473011418820847.
2. Myerson MS. Adult acquired flatfoot deformity: treatment of dysfunction of the posterior tibial tendon. Instr Course Lect 1997;46:393–405.
3. Thordarson DB, Schmotzer H, Chon J, et al. Dynamic support of the human longitudinal arch. a biomechanical evaluation. Clin Orthop Relat Res 1995;316: 165–72.
4. Thordarson DB, Schmotzer H, Chon J. Reconstruction with tenodesis in an adult flatfoot model. a biomechanical evaluation of four methods. J Bone Joint Surg Am 1995;77:1557–64.
5. Robberecht J, Shah DS, Taylan O, et al. The role of medial ligaments and tibialis posterior in stabilising the medial longitudinal foot arch: a cadaveric gait simulator study. Foot Ankle Surg 2021;28(7):906–11.
6. Lee MS, Vanore JV, Thomas JL, et al. Diagnosis and treatment of adult flatfoot. J Foot Ankle Surg 2005;44:78–113.
7. Deland JT. Adult-acquired flatfoot deformity. J Am Acad Orthop Surg 2008;16: 399–406.
8. Jackson JB 3rd, Pacana MJ, Gonzalez TA. Adult acquired flatfoot deformity. J Am Acad Orthop Surg 2022;30(1):e6–16.
9. Johnson KA, Strom DE. Tibialis posterior tendon dysfunction. Clin Orthop Relat Res 1989;(239):196–206.
10. Bluman EM, Title CI, Myerson MS. Posterior tibial tendon rupture: a refined classification system. Foot Ankle Clin 2007;12:233–49.
11. Pasapula C, Devany A, Fischer NC, et al. The resistance to failure of spring ligament reconstruction. Foot (Edinb) 2017;33:29–34.

12. Rule J, Yao L, Seeger LL. Spring ligament of the ankle: normal MR anatomy. AJR Am J Roentgenol 1993;161(6):1241–4.
13. Kelly M, Masqoodi N, Vasconcellos D, et al. Spring ligament tear decreases static stability of the ankle joint. Clin Biomech (Bristol, Avon) 2019;61:79–83.
14. Bastias GF, Dalmau-Pastor M, Astudillo C, et al. Spring ligament instability. Foot Ankle Clin 2018;23(4):659–78.
15. Lin YC, Kwon JY, Ghorbanhoseini M, et al. The hindfoot arch: what role does the imager play? Radiol Clin North Am 2016;54(5):951–68.
16. Pasapula C, Devany A, Magan A, et al. Neutral heel lateral push test: the first clinical examination of spring ligament integrity. Foot (Edinb) 2015;25(2):69–74.
17. Davis WH, Sobel M, DiCarlo EF, et al. Gross, histological, and microvascular anatomy and biomechanical testing of the spring ligament complex. Foot Ankle Int 1996;17(2):95–102.
18. Masaragian HJ, Massetti S, Perin F, et al. Flatfoot deformity due to isolated spring ligament injury. J Foot Ankle Surg 2020;59(3):469–78.
19. Cifuentes-De la Portilla C, Pasapula C, Larrainzar-Garijo R, et al. Finite element analysis of secondary effect of midfoot fusions on the spring ligament in the management of adult acquired flatfoot. Clin Biomech (Bristol, Avon) 2020;76:105018.
20. Lui TH. Endoscopic repair of the superficial deltoid ligament and spring ligament. Arthrosc Tech 2016;5(3):e621–5.
21. Nery C, Lemos AVKC, Raduan F, et al. Combined spring and deltoid ligament repair in adult-acquired flatfoot. Foot Ankle Int 2018;39(8):903–7.
22. Malakoutikhah H, Madenci E, Latt LD. The contribution of the ligaments in progressive collapsing foot deformity: a comprehensive computational study. J Orthop Res 2022;40(9):2209–21.
23. Van Boerum DH, Sangeorzan BJ. Biomechanics and pathophysiology of flat foot. Foot Ankle Clin 2003;8(3):419–30.
24. Myerson MS, Thordarson DB, Johnson JE, et al. Classification and nomenclature: progressive collapsing foot deformity. Foot Ankle Int 2020;41(10):1271–6.
25. Aynardi MC, Saloky K, Roush EP, et al. Biomechanical evaluation of spring ligament augmentation with the fibertape device in a cadaveric flatfoot model. Foot Ankle Int 2019;40(5):596–602.
26. Lui TH. Arthroscopic repair of superomedial spring ligament by talonavicular arthroscopy. Arthrosc Tech 2017;6(1):e31–5.
27. Oburu E, Myerson MS. Deltoid ligament repair in flatfoot deformity. Foot Ankle Clin 2017;22(3):503–14.
28. Cifuentes-De la Portilla C, Larrainzar-Garijo R, Bayod J. Analysis of the main passive soft tissues associated with adult acquired flatfoot deformity development: a computational modeling approach. J Biomech 2019;84:183–90.
29. Cifuentes-De la Portilla C, Larrainzar-Garijo R, Bayod J. Analysis of biomechanical stresses caused by hindfoot joint arthrodesis in the treatment of adult acquired flatfoot deformity: a finite element study. Foot Ankle Surg 2020;26(4):412–20.
30. Niu W, Tang T, Zhang M, et al. An in vitro and finite element study of load redistribution in the midfoot. Sci China Life Sci 2014;57(12):1191–6.
31. Deland JT, de Asla RJ, Sung IH, et al. Posterior tibial tendon insufficiency: which ligaments are involved? Foot Ankle Int 2005;26(6):427–35.
32. Tryfonidis M, Jackson W, Mansour R, et al. Acquired adult flat foot due to isolated plantar calcaneonavicular (spring) ligament insufficiency with a normal tibialis posterior tendon. Foot Ankle Surg 2008;14(2):89–95.

33. Flores DV, Mejía Gómez C, Fernández Hernando M, et al. Adult acquired flatfoot deformity: anatomy, biomechanics, staging, and imaging findings. Radiographics 2019;39(5):1437–60.

34. Cheung JT, Zhang M, An KN. Effects of plantar fascia stiffness on the biomechanical responses of the ankle-foot complex. Clin Biomech (Bristol, Avon) 2004; 19(8):839–46.

35. Choi K, Lee S, Otis JC, et al. Anatomical reconstruction of the spring ligament using peroneus longus tendon graft. Foot Ankle Int 2003;24(5):430–6.

36. Ellis SJ, Williams BR, Wagshul AD, et al. Deltoid ligament reconstruction with peroneus longus autograft in flatfoot deformity. Foot Ankle Int 2010;31(9):781–9.

37. Grunfeld R, Oh I, Flemister S, et al. Reconstruction of the deltoid spring ligament. Tech Foot Ankle Surg 2016;15:39–46.

38. Raikin SM, Rogero RG, Raikin J, et al. Outcomes of 2B adult acquired flatfoot deformity correction in patients with and without spring ligament tear. Foot Ankle Int 2021;42(12):1517–24.

39. Brodell JD, MacDonald A, Perkins JA, et al. Deltoidspring ligament reconstruction in adult acquired flatfoot deformity with medial peritalar instability. Foot Ankle Int 2019;40:753–61.

40. Fogleman JA, Kreulen CD, Sarcon AK, et al. Augmented spring ligament repair in pes planovalgus reconstruction. J Foot Ankle Surg 2021;60(6):1212–6.

41. Tang CYK, Ng KH. A valuable option: clinical and radiological outcomes of braided suture tape system augmentation for spring ligament repair in flexible flatfoot. Foot (Edinb) 2020;45:101685.

42. Krautmann K, Kadakia AR. Spring and deltoid ligament insufficiency in the setting of progressive collapsing foot deformity. an update on diagnosis and management. Foot Ankle Clin 2021;26(3):577–90.

43. Acevedo J, Vora A. Anatomical reconstruction of the spring ligament complex: "internal brace" augmentation. Foot Ankle Spec 2013;6(6):441–5.

44. MacDonald A, Ciufo D, Vess E, et al. Peritalar kinematics with combined deltoid-spring ligament reconstruction in simulated advanced adult acquired flatfoot deformity. Foot Ankle Int 2020;41(9):1149–57.

Double versus Triple Arthrodesis for Flatfoot Deformity: When, Why, and How?

Patrick R. Burns, DPM[a],*, Nicholas S. Powers, DPM[b]

KEYWORDS

• Triple arthrodesis • Double arthrodesis • Flatfoot • Foot surgery

KEY POINTS

• Arthrodesis remains a consistent way to address rigid flatfoot deformity that can not be corrected with tendon transfers or osteotomies.
• Outcomes and discussion continue with arthrodesis of the talonavicular, subtalar and calcanealcuboid joints in double versus triple arthrodesis.

Flatfoot treatment is an important and often revisited topic for the foot and ankle surgeon. We continue to gain understanding of the deformity, the biomechanics, our ability to intervene, and the long-term effects of treatment. Techniques continue to evolve with this improved understanding, but arthrodesis remains a consistent, reliable way to address flatfoot, particularly in severe arthritic change and with more difficult deformities. Although arthrodesis for flatfoot has been around for many years, we still strive to improve results with modified surgical approaches, changing fixation techniques, and adjuncts to arthrodesis to fine-tune and improve outcomes. This review will evaluate some of the current debate and discussion regarding fusion of the talonavicular joint (TNJ), subtalar joint (STJ), and calcaneal cuboid joint (CCJ) or triple arthrodesis (TA) versus fusion of the TNJ and STJ or double arthrodesis (DA).

Arthrodesis has been a reliable and mainstay surgical treatment to address flatfoot deformities.[1–5] There are several indications for arthrodesis in flatfoot reconstruction that are similar for both TA and DA procedures. The most obvious is a deformity with arthritic components to the rearfoot joints. As we have no implant arthroplasty for the rearfoot joints, arthrodesis remains the treatment of choice. Secondly, some deformities are too severe to be corrected with osteotomies or tendon transfers alone and thus require arthrodesis for adequate correction. Patient demographics, including

[a] University of Pittsburgh School of Medicine, University of Pittsburgh Physicians, Comprehensive Foot & Ankle Center, 1515 Locust Street #350, Pittsburgh, PA 15219, USA; [b] Department of Orthopaedic Surgery, Atrium Health Wake Forest Baptist, Wake Forest University School of Medicine, Medical Center Boulevard, Winston-Salem, NC 27157, USA
* Corresponding author.
E-mail address: burnsp@upmc.edu

Clin Podiatr Med Surg 40 (2023) 315–332
https://doi.org/10.1016/j.cpm.2022.11.009
0891-8422/23/© 2022 Elsevier Inc. All rights reserved.

age and weight, should also be considered during procedure selection.[6,7] A geriatric patient with a typical, flexible Stage 2 posterior tibial tendon dysfunction and acquired flatfoot has been shown to have good short-term outcomes with osteotomies and tendon transfers.[8] However, the longevity of such procedures has not been established nor has it been compared directly to TA or DA procedures. Likewise, transferring a tendon and performing osteotomies on an obese or super-obese patient may not hold up or perform as anticipated. As such, in many cases, arthrodesis may be a more predictable and robust choice.[7] Finally, TA and DA procedures may be indicated in cases of revision flatfoot surgery. They are certainly warranted in revision arthrodesis, but may be the only remaining option if tendon transfers and osteotomies have already been performed.

Once a surgeon has chosen to perform either the TA or DA procedures, the joints are exposed and prepared for arthrodesis. The respective joints are debrided of cartilage according to surgeon's preference, often using a combination of osteotomes, curettes, and powered burrs. The deformity is then reduced and fixated. For the long standing, rigid, or severe deformities the surgeon may also perform osteotomies in conjunction with standard joint preparation to adequately reduce the deformities.[9,10] Performing simultaneous bone cuts and osteotomies at the time of joint preparation allows the surgeon to correct even the most severe deformities and maintain high patient-reported outcomes.

TRIPLE VERSUS DOUBLE

Once the decision is made to perform an arthrodesis procedure for a flatfoot deformity, the next questions is when and why would a surgeon choose TA over DA or vice versa? There are many factors involved in making the decision to perform an arthrodesis procedure. Some of these factors include the previously mentioned age, weight, severity of deformity, flexibility of deformity, the patient's medical history, and history of prior surgery.[11–13] With all the information, a decision can then be made as to which joints to include. Essentially, at this point the question is whether or not to include the CCJ into the fusion mass. The surgeon ultimately has to decide if the benefits of including the CCJ in the procedure outweigh the risk of the added procedure.

From a biomechanical standpoint, the three joints being discussed function to assist in the foot's ability to accommodate to surfaces. The rearfoot joints can lock and limit motion, providing a rigid lever for propulsion but also unlock to accommodate impact and allow motion.[14] The interplay of these joints is complicated and the source of many of the deformities and pathology associated with flatfoot. Understanding these joints and how to manipulate their interaction is the basis of flatfoot surgical intervention. The CCJ arthrodesis has been shown to have the least influence of the three joints on overall hindfoot motion.[15] The landmark article by Astion and colleagues[16] revealed that simulated arthrodesis of the CCJ allowed 67% of the original TNJ motion and 92% of the original STJ motion in five cadaveric feet. The TNJ and STJ provide most of the motion through the rearfoot, so including the CCJ in the arthrodesis provides little additional restriction of abnormal motion. Wulker and colleagues[17] confirmed that fusion of the CCJ had no significant influence on remaining hindfoot motion and that any arthrodesis including the TNJ almost completely eliminated motion at the CCJ. On the contrary, maintaining those few degrees from the CCJ could actually help postoperatively by allowing for some accommodation along the lateral column and therefore limiting lateral column symptoms seen in the more standard TA.[18,19]

One of the most common indications for either triple or DA includes addressing the sequelae of posterior tibial tendon dysfunction. Arthrodesis can correct the resultant deformities but can also significantly limit the excursion of the posterior tibial tendon. Limiting the overall movement of the diseased tendon may aid in pain relief. But adding the CCJ into the arthrodesis seems to have minimal effect on this as well which again would call into question the need to include it for posterior tibial tendon pain relief. The excursion of the posterior tibial tendon was affected significantly in the Astion and colleagues[16] article to only 25% of its original movement anytime the TNJ was included. With the small number of specimens, the CCJ did not produce numbers to evaluate but would appear to have limited ability to provide additional restriction on the posterior tibial tendon excursion. As the TNJ arthrodesis seems to be the major player in restricting range of motion and posterior tibial tendon excursion, pain relief is presumably similar for both triple and DA.[20]

Another consideration for choosing between triple and DA is the calcaneocuboid joint itself. If the deformity to be addressed includes arthritis, including the CCJ into the arthrodesis should improve pain outcomes. But studies show comparable pain outcome results between TA and DA. In fact, Berlet and colleagues[18] showed in a report of 20 DA patients, radiographic signs of arthritis seemed to improve or reverse. These findings included a more normal joint contour, increased joint space to the CCJ, and less sclerosis at mean follow of 9.2 months. In their discussion, considerations for these improvements include effects from distraction arthrodiastasis of the CCJ, similar to what has been reported in the ankle arthritis literature.[21] Distracting an arthritic joint may have some reparative qualities. With the flatfoot correction, the calcaneal cuboid abduction angle and lateral column impingement is addressed and the CCJ is distracted or opened (**Fig. 1**). The deformity correction is stable through the TNJ and STJ arthrodesis, allowing for correction and pain relief while retaining lateral column motion and improving the lateral column length.[22] This removes pressure along the lateral column but may be of limited use if the CCJ is already significantly arthritic.[3]

As the primary indication for TA and DA discussed within this article is flatfoot deformity, it is worth discussing lateral column deformity as well. One of the common findings in flatfoot deformity is a shortened lateral column. This is evident in radiographic changes in the transverse plane, such as the calcaneal cuboid abduction angle on the anterior-posterior projection of the foot. Lateral column length is frequently addressed with procedures such as the Evans osteotomy and even CCJ distraction arthrodesis.[23–25] But these are typically earlier or less severe flatfoot deformities. When rearfoot arthrodesis is considered, the correction is done through the fusion itself. In a traditional TA the CCJ is usually prepared and fixed in situ. For many deformities, the surgeon has corrected the forefoot abduction through adducting the TNJ, which then leaves a deficit or gap laterally. To achieve a TA, the midfoot and forefoot then have to be brought back to abduction to have the CCJ surface approximate for fusion. This counteracts the original reduction and surgical plan, making this a counterproductive procedure for many surgeons. The other option is to leave the CCJ distracted and then fill the void with bone graft (**Fig. 2**). Of course, doing this is more complicated, adds time to the operation, and may prove to be more difficult to heal. Bone graft interposed to the CCJ then has to incorporate between two subchondral bone surfaces and can have a high complication and nonunion rate.[24,25] In performing a DA, the medial reduction and fixation corrects the flatfoot deformity, whereas the CCJ would be distracted. This offers biomechanical advantages previously mentioned and avoids the need to heal and incorporate an interpositional bone graft.

In addition to all of the previously mentioned considerations between TA and DA, the surgeon should also consider operating room time. It is reasonable to assume that a

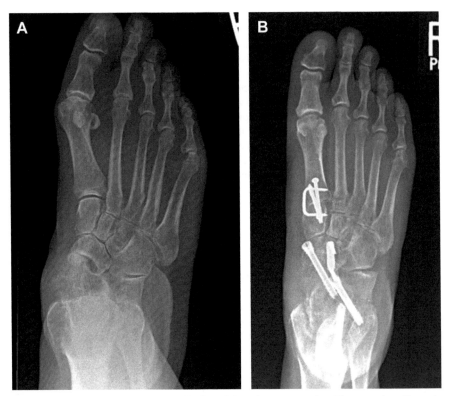

Fig. 1. Radiographs or preoperative flatfoot (*A*) and postoperative (*B*) correction. Note the distracted CCJ and more linear lateral column.

single incision approach or smaller incisions would be quicker with less time for dissection and for wound closure. Similarly, time for application of fixation should be quicker for two joints versus three, particularly when considering interpositional grafting at the CCJ. In fact, studies have shown differences between TA and DA surgical times.[13,26,27] As long as the outcomes are similar in terms of deformity correction, overall pain control, and patient satisfaction, then this could be a critical argument. In a world of increasing efficiency, limited operating room availability, and staffing shortages in health care, operating times warrant serious consideration. If there is no real benefit found to including the CCJ, then this may be the most useful argument against including it in the construct.

INCISION APPROACHES

In addition to considering the underlying deformity and arthritic changes, a surgeon must consider surgical approaches and the risks associated with soft tissue injuries. Wound healing problems have been reported in up to one-third of the patients undergoing major reconstruction and arthrodesis for flatfoot.[25] Traditional TA is done through two incisions.[28,29] The first is the classic lateral sinus tarsi incision for the STJ and CCJ that runs from the tip of the fibula to the base of the fourth metatarsal (**Fig. 3**). Dissection through this area allows access to the STJ after removing the contents of the sinus tarsi, as well as the CCJ after the extensor digitorum brevis muscle belly is reflected. The second incision is to gain access to the TNJ. There are two

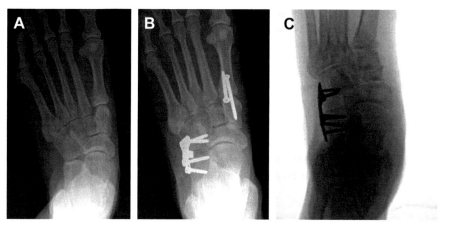

Fig. 2. Typical abducted flatfoot on AP radiograph (*A*) once corrected leaving a gap at the CCJ. Opening wedge plates (*B*) and bone graft (*C*) are ways to help manage this void during CCJ distraction arthrodesis.

common approaches to the TNJ that can be used. Each has its own advantages which will be discussed. In recent years, other approaches have been explored as well including a single lateral incision and arthroscopy.[30,31]

When considering surgical incisions, the medial approach to the TNJ and STJ with either TA or DA warrant special consideration. In particular, there are concerns about proximal dissection along the medial incision near the medial malleolus and medial

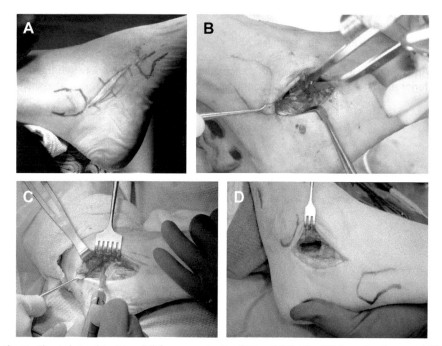

Fig. 3. Classic lateral incision (*A*) for access to the STJ and CCJ. The STJ is easily distracted (*B*) and prepared (*C, D*) with this incision.

talus (**Fig. 4**). The deltoid ligament is often disrupted to gain full access to the STJ and to allow enough access for joint preparation. Portions of the deltoid can be compromised and the surgeon must understand the local anatomy around the more proximal medial structures within that approach to limit transection of the deltoid ligament. For many flatfoot patients undergoing arthrodesis, there may already be compromise to the medial soft tissue structures from years of medial column collapse and stress. The posterior tibial tendon for flatfoot has not been performing active support of the medial column sufficiently, adding strain to the static support structures like the deltoid ligament. Further dissection and transection of portions of the deltoid during the medial surgical approach can further compromise the support, potentially contributing to ankle valgus postoperatively.[31] Another issue during the single medial approach to TA or DA, may be an injury to the deltoid artery, artery of the tarsal canal and artery of the tarsal sinus in cadaver studies.[32,33] It is well known that the medial aspect of the talus and the talar body would have potential consequences in blood supply and possible fusion rates if there is significant dissection through the deltoid ligament. The single medial approach can have effects on both the deltoid branches but also then the sinus tarsi circulation as that is typically debrided and evacuated as well. The more traditional two incision approaches may violate the artery of the tarsal sinus but medial arterial supply is typically not disturbed.

The traditional medial approach for isolated TNJ preparation is over the medial aspect of the joint at the interval between the tibialis posterior and tibialis anterior tendons (**Fig. 5**). This incision begins near the tip of the medial malleolus and runs distal to the navicular cuneiform joint. This is similar to the medial approach for both TNJ and STJ, but requires less proximal dissection. For some, this is preferred as it gives access to the posterior tibial tendon itself for repair or excision depending on surgeon preference and surgical needs. There may be some limitations in regard to the complete TNJ exposure and difficulty with cartilage removal laterally.[34] From a fixation standpoint, there may be some limitations as well. The whole dorsal surface is unable to effectively be accessed directly, so fixation to secure this section of the joint may be more difficult to apply or may necessitate percutaneous fixation.

An alternative incision placement to access the TNJ is dorsally between the tibialis anterior and the extensor hallucis longus tendons (**Fig. 6**). This is a safe interval that

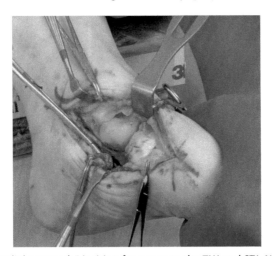

Fig. 4. Typical "medial approach" incision for access to the TNJ and STJ. Note the dissection required and possible injury to deltoid ligament.

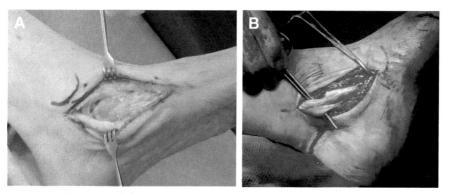

Fig. 5. More limited medial incision for access to the TNJ (A) with the talar head noted in the wound. The posterior tibial tendon is directly visualization with this incision (B) and can be excised or mobilized if needed.

gives dorsal access to the whole TNJ for joint preparation. Joint preparation may be more complete[35] and fixation of the dorsal surface and body of the navicular and TNJ may be more manageable. This approach gives a large area for plates, screws, and staples. However, it may also require percutaneous fixation, particularly for surgeons who prefer a compression screw from the navicular tuberosity. Another con for this dorsal incision is that you cannot access the other rearfoot joints. If the goal is to do a TA or DA through a single incision, then the dorsal approach to the TNJ is not appropriate.

Finally, a single lateral incision to expose all three joints has been proposed. The TNJ is accessed through the same lateral sinus tarsi incision using bone retractors. Ohly and colleagues[30], reported on 30 patients undergoing TA with this approach. Eleven were classified as posterior tibial tendon dysfunction, but the other etiologies of "acquired flatfoot" included rheumatoid arthritis, osteoarthritis, and ankylosing spondylitis. All had the single lateral incision with preparation of the joints by high-speed burr with allograft application. In their series, there was only one wound complication requiring vacuum-assisted closure and two patients with rheumatoid arthritis that had progression to pantalar at 16 and 39 months postoperatively. There were

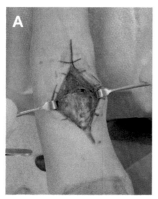
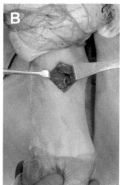
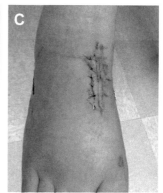

Fig. 6. Dorsal approach to the TNJ (A, C) which allows more direct fixation of the body, dorsal and lateral aspect of the joint (B).

no issues with bone union in this study but there have been questions about joint preparation with this approach. The TNJ may not be completely accessible. This study revealed no issue with access to the whole TNJ and had no issues with union; however, there are studies that estimate only 38% of the TNJ can be accessed with this single lateral incision.[35]

The lateral sinus tarsi incision may be more concerning when considering more severe and rigid flatfoot deformities. One issue is the removal of the soft tissue within the sinus tarsi which then limits the amount of tissue available for coverage and closure. The other concern is the tension applied to the incision after closure. With the often longstanding nature of the flatfoot deformity, the lateral soft tissue has contracted over time with a valgus heel and forefoot abduction. Once the deformity is corrected with boney procedures, the lateral skin closure is then placed under tension with a more rectus foot. Limited soft tissue and tissue under tension after deformity correction is hypothesized as a cause of wound complications. Because of these concerns, some surgeons choose to avoid the lateral incision altogether.[13,31,36–38] To address these concerns, many surgeons who prefer the lateral incision attempt to limit the incision length, minimize trauma and handling of the soft tissue, and optimize operating time. In the case of DA, the need for a longer incision and extensive dissection is negated with no distal joint exposure necessary. With no need to expose the CCJ, the muscle belly of the extensor digitorum brevis is kept in place, limiting the dissection and trauma to local soft tissue. There is also no need for distal fixation which minimizes soft tissue handling and decreases the overall time in the operating room.

An alternative for STJ and CCJ preparation and deformity correction is the medial approach (**Fig. 7**). This was described by Jeng and colleagues,[36] reporting good results on TA using this approach in 17 patients. The technique was used because of the concerns regarding wound complications with the lateral soft tissue due to preoperative deformity. They reported 15 of 17 achieving arthrodesis of all three joints, and only two having pseudoarthrosis of the CCJ which was asymptomatic. In the Jeng article, all three joints were accessed with the single medial approach however many have used this same approach to achieve a DA instead.[38] For either TA or DA, the incision is along the medial foot between the tibialis anterior tendon and posterior tibial tendon. It begins at the tip of the medial malleolus and is extended distal, coursing over the TNJ. With the incision deepened, the TNJ is accessed first. With further dissection, the STJ and even the CCJ can be reached deep to the posterior tibial tendon.[37,39] Depending on pathology and surgeon preference, the posterior tibial tendon can be excised, debrided or retracted superior to gain access to the interosseous ligaments and the deeper remaining joints. This approach has become attractive to some surgeons performing either TA or DA to address flatfoot deformities.[40] In recent studies, however, there has been some cause for concern regarding this

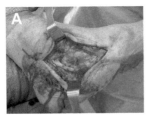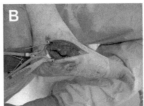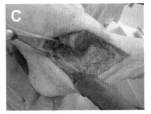

Fig. 7. Further example of a medial approach to the TNJ, STJ, and CCJ. Note the soft tissue dissection needed (*A, B*) with possible violation of the deltoid ligament. All three joints can be accessed (*C*) with this approach.

technique including incomplete correction and issues accessing the whole joint sur-faces.[40] As mentioned earlier, proximal dissection may compromise the deltoid liga-ment. Compromising the deltoid ligament, in particular the deep portions, gives rise to concern for continued or progressive ankle valgus following arthrodesis.[41] The arte-rial and blood supply concerns have been discussed when sacrificing the deltoid as well which may increase chances for nonunion.[32,33]

Finally, arthroscopic approaches have been described with emphasis on limiting extensive soft tissue dissection.[42,43] First described by Lui and colleagues[42], an arthroscope is used with either two, three, or four portals (**Fig. 8**). Initially, it was described with a 2.7 mm arthroscope; however, some authors use a 4.0 mm scope. Like any arthroscopic technique, there is a learning curve, particularly with smaller joints, but in recent years the approach has been shown to address complex defor-mities successfully and the number of portals has become fewer. One recent study showed good outcomes with just two sinus tarsi incisions to access all joints for either for a TA or DA.[44] Arthroscopic indications primarily include conditions causing poor skin quality or trauma with old skin incisions, whereas contraindications would include rigid deformities or the need for bone grafting.

FIXATION

A variety of options are available for the foot and ankle surgeon to achieve rigid fixation after the flatfoot deformity has been corrected. Fixation selections include solid and cannulated screws of varying sizes, as well as many headless designs. There are stan-dard and anatomic plates with cortical and locking designs as well as an increasing variety of standard and compression staples. These improvements in technology have given the surgeon the ability to realize more robust fixation in particular with the limited size and bone available in the hindfoot. External fixation has been described as well but should be limited to revision or other circumstances. In one study by Talarico and colleagues[45], 87 patients had TA with external fixation and arched wire for compression. All patients were partial weight bearing from the first postoperative week and 97% achieved fusion. Although favorable union rates,

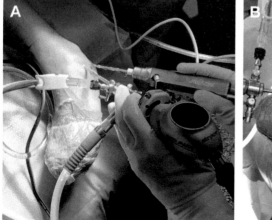
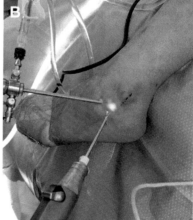

Fig. 8. Typical STJ access for arthroscopic preparation of the STJ (*A, B*). The author uses two incisions with the patient in a lateral position and the foot hanging off a bump for better access.

complications included 36% with one or more pin site complications and 10% had wound healing complications.

Screws are the mainstay of fixation with cannulated varieties being the most common. Cannulated screws now come in many different sizes and the guide wires can act as provisional fixation. Smaller sizes give the ability to place multiple screws and screws in orientations that may not have been possible with the limited larger cannulated screws years ago. The cannulation also allows for proper positioning not only of the deformity but the screws themselves to achieve the best possible construct.

Plate design and technology has allowed a significant growth in what is available for the foot and ankle surgeon. Smaller screws have allowed for smaller, more anatomic plates increasing fixation options. Most plates are now locking technology as well, adding to the stability in small, irregular anatomic locations like the rearfoot.

Staples have made a recurrence in recent years with improvements in materials and compression characteristics. Many companies today offer differing sizes and materials that have "memory" providing continuous compression.[46] This continuous compression may be beneficial when considering potential for bone resorption at arthrodesis sites. Although screws and plates will lose their ability to maintain compression with resorption, continuous compression staples provide some ability to maintain compression across the joint. In addition, staples may generate compression more evenly across a joint which is otherwise difficult to access without compromising adjacent bones or joints with more traditional screw fixation, particularly at the TNJ and CCJ. Most are predrilled and offer guides that make them a quick, simple form of fixation whether alone or as an adjunct. The ease of staple placement may reduce operative times as well. Cadaveric studies have shown no difference in strength between staples and screws for TA.[47,48]

The most common construct for the STJ seems to be two screws with placement in a divergent fashion (**Fig. 9**). Although one versus two screws has not shown statistical significance in fusion outcomes, two screws have been shown to have greater torsional stiffness compared with a single screw or even two placed in a parallel fashion.[49–52] Additional studies have shown a screw for the STJ placed from dorsal to plantar has greater pull-out strength than those placed from plantar to dorsal[53] (**Fig. 10**). Screws placed from the plantar calcaneal tuberosity also have a higher chance of prominence and irritation necessitating removal.[50] With the rising popularity of headless compression designs, prominence and irritation from screw heads may become less of a surgical concern though. Other considerations for orientation of STJ screws are thread length. From dorsal to plantar, there is frequently the opportunity to use the longer thread pattern of most hardware companies adding to fixation. From plantar to dorsal, the talar body and neck are shallower so only short thread patterns can be used.[53] Finally, there are other configurations reported as surgeons look

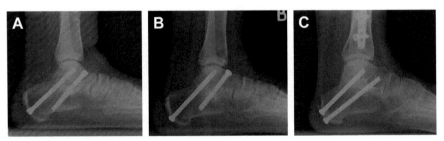

Fig. 9. Common STJ fixation with opposing headless screws (*A*) and headed screws (*B*). Two screws can also be placed from plantar to dorsal in a divergent manner (*C*).

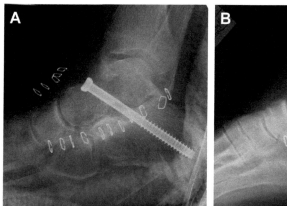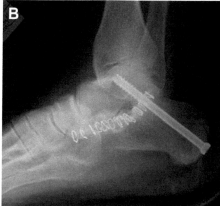

Fig. 10. Single screw fixation for the STJ. Note the ability to use a long thread pattern when the screw is placed from dorsal to plantar (*A*) and the short thread pattern when the screw are placed from the plantar aspect (*B*).

to achieve stability in multiple planes but limit the amount of actual joint destroyed by fixation. One such idea described by Boffeli and colleagues[54] includes an augmentation with a plantar to dorsal STJ screw with a second screw passed from the lateral plantar aspect of the anterior calcaneus to the talar neck dorsally. This screw acts as a positional screw while allowing the maximum amount of raw bone surface for fusion without the disruption of multiple screws.

The TNJ most often has primary fixation by a screw retrograde from the navicular tuberosity into the body of the talus. With the advent of smaller screws, plates, and staples augmenting TNJ fixation has become common (**Fig. 11**). Many add a plate or staple; however, in one study by Vacketta and colleagues,[55] four types of TNJ fixation were retrospectively evaluated. During DA, there was a total of 16.2% nonunion rate in their 105 patients. Their three-screw group for TNJ fixation had the lowest nonunion rate of 2.4%. They were placed medial at the tuberosity, the central body and then lateral body from distal to proximal (**Fig. 12**). Their two-screw cohort had a 33.3% nonunion rate, a single screw plus a plate had a 16.0% nonunion rate and finally their two-screw plus plate construct had a 29.4% nonunion rate. To increase stability and aid in fusion rates, alternatives and adjuncts have been proposed as well. An augmenting "naviculocalcaneal" screw during DA in a cadaveric study described by Kiesau and colleagues[56] improved mean bending stiffness in all directions tested. Ten cadavers had two 4.5 mm cannulated screws placed across the TNJ. Testing was performed and then the same specimens had a third screw placed from the lateral portion of the navicular into the calcaneus with the same four directions tested. Adding the "naviculocalcaneal" screw significantly improved performance of the construct leading to the conclusion this could aid in fusion rates.

If a decision has been made to include the CCJ and perform a more traditional TA, a single screw has been described.[57] The orientation can be difficult and achieving stable compression perpendicular to the fusion site is difficult with the size and shape of the bones and joint. A screw can be placed from the anterior process into the cuboid but the angle does not allow for strong perpendicular compression. To achieve perpendicular, a screw can be placed from the posterior tuberosity of the calcaneus into the cuboid, but that can be technically difficult and requires a long screw with short thread pattern (**Fig. 13**). To address these shortcomings, staples and locking

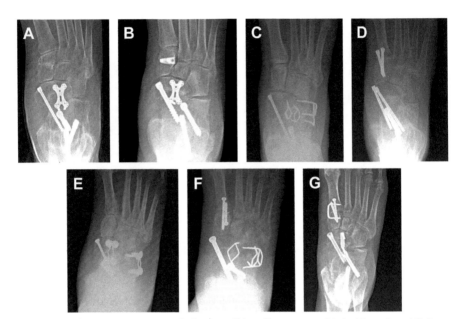

Fig. 11. TNJ fixation variations including small headless screw with locking plate (*A*), large headless screw with locking plate (*B*), one small headless screw (*C*), two small headless screws (*D*), a headed screw with a compression plate (*E*), one large headed screw and compression staple (*F*), and one large headless screw with compression staple (*G*).

plates have been used. The advent of compression staples and locking technology of small anatomic plates has allowed for technically easier application and possibly increased strength. A study of five matched pairs of cadavers found a single oblique screw construct failed with less force and achieved less stiffness compared with a compression locking plate placed on the lateral surface of the CCJ.[58]

And finally, there may be circumstances to use external fixation as either primary or as a revision surgery. There are systems to allow foot and ankle surgeons to place pins through the rearfoot and use unilateral compression devices to achieve fusion (**Fig. 14**). More common would be the use of circular multiplane fixators as either

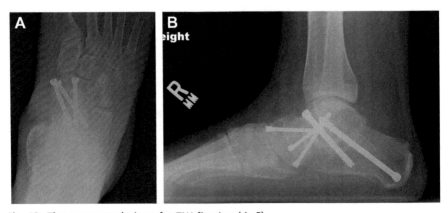

Fig. 12. Three screw technique for TNJ fixation (*A, B*).

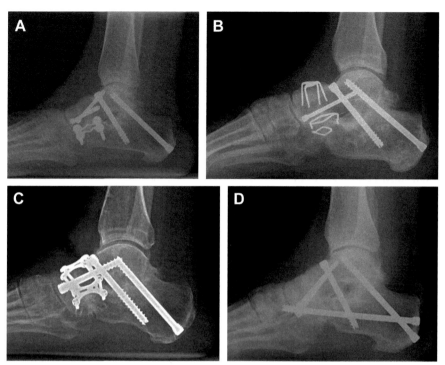

Fig. 13. Fixation for the CCJ including compression plate (*A*), compression staples (*B*), single locking plate (*C*), and screw fixation from posterior (*D*).

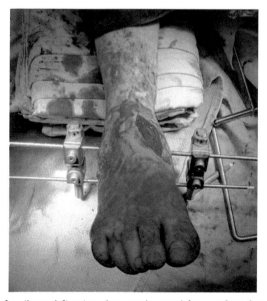

Fig. 14. Example of unilateral fixation that can be used for rearfoot fusions.

augmentation or as primary hardware.[45] When used as primary fixation, the skinny wires are tensioned after bending or "walking" them along the external fixator. The joints to be fused are prepared in the standard fashion, and reduction is held with smooth Kirschner wires. The external fixator is applied in the standard fashion with attention being drawn to the fixation of the talus, navicular, cuboid and calcaneus. Wires through the talus, navicular, and cuboid will be used to compress the associated joints. These wires are pulled perpendicular to their corresponding joints and then have a gentle bow before attaching to the frame. This is the "bent wire" technique (**Fig. 15**). When tension is then applied the wire attempts to straighten. This causes compression against the corresponding bone and proximal component. For example, the talus wire through the neck of the talus is placed lateral to medial, and is then "bent" down and back to the foot plate where it is connected. As tension is applied to the wire, this creates a force against the calcaneus and compresses the STJ. Likewise, wires through the navicular and cuboid are walked posterior on the fixator before tension is applied. These wires then compress the TNJ and CCJ. The fixator is kept in place until union is seen and then removed.

FINAL DISCUSSION

The decision to perform arthrodesis for flatfoot deformity has had relatively consistent indications over the years and has been shown to be a mainstay of treatment which has withstood the test of time. However, choosing between TA and DA procedures for flatfoot deformity has been debated for a number of reasons outlined in the current

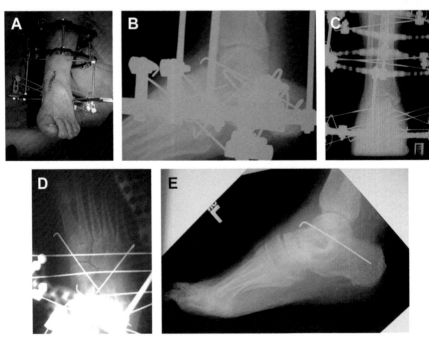

Fig. 15. The use of circular external fixation for TA (*A*). Wires through the talus, navicular, and cuboid can be "walked" before being connected and tensioned to create the "bent wire" technique of compression. As the wire is tensioned, it attempt to straighten creating force against the proximal segment (*B–D*). Note the Kwire that remains which was used for temporary fixation during frame application with good fusion (*E*).

article. Although the traditional TA has shown favorable outcomes time and again, the DA has gained more and more popularity in recent years. The TA addresses the three joint complex directly; however, the utility of including the CCJ has been called into question, even in the setting of advanced degenerative changes of the CCJ.

It is generally the authors' preference to perform a DA through a dual incision approach over the traditional TA. The lateral approach to the STJ from the distal tip of the fibula toward the fourth metatarsal base is used. This minimizes distal dissection and soft tissue handling laterally at the CCJ while avoiding potential deltoid ligament and arterial compromise with the proximal medial dissection required with a single medial approach to DA. In addition, it avoids need for interpositional grafting at the CCJ and ultimately decreases risk of CCJ nonunion while maintaining the motion and adaptation of the lateral column. Fixation is typically performed with two cannulated screws across the posterior facet of the STJ in a divergent fashion. One screw is placed from posterior to anterior, whereas the other is placed from anterior to posterior, starting on the talar neck. This allows for increased divergence and increased thread length with the anterior-to-posterior screw placement. The preferred approach to the TNJ is with a dorsal incisional approach between the tibialis anterior and extensor hallucis longus tendons. This provides good joint exposure while allowing complete access to the dorsal joint for robust fixation. Fixation typically involves a single cannulated screw from the navicular tuberosity through a percutaneous incision as well as dorsal lateral fixation either with a locking plate or staple construct in an attempt to provide the evenest compression and stability across a deep and irregularly shaped joint.

Whether a surgeon chooses to perform TA or DA, he or she must consider all of the variables including patient-specific risks for healing soft tissue and osseous procedures, a variety of incisional approaches, and an increasing number and variety of fixation options. In doing so, he or she should attempt to provide the best patient-centered outcomes while minimizing the risks of interventions. Regardless of a surgeon's preference, there is plenty of literature to support good outcomes with both procedures. However, there is limited evidence comparing the procedures directly, partly owing to the significant heterogeneity of indications, approaches, and fixation options. As such, the debate between TA and DA for flatfoot deformity will likely continue into the foreseeable future.

CLINICS CARE POINTS

- Double verus triple arthrodesis continues to be a point of discussion among surgeons.
- Patient specific risks, incisional approach and fixation are points of consideration when deciding Double versus triple arthrodesis.

REFERENCES

1. Coetzee JC, Castro MD. The indications and biomechanical rationale for various hindfoot procedures in the treatment of posterior tibialis tendon dysfunction. Foot Ankle Clin 2003;8(3):453–9.
2. Meehan RE, Brage M. Adult acquired flat foot deformity: clinical and radiographic examination. Foot Ankle Clin 2003;8(3):431–52.
3. Erard MUE, Sheean MAJ, Sangeorzan BJ. Triple arthrodesis for adult-acquired flatfoot deformity. Foot Ankle Orthop 2019;4(3):1–12.

4. Gobbo DKP, Severino NR, Ferreira RC. What is the prognosis of triple arthrodesis in the treatment of adult acquired flatfoot deformity (AAFD)? Rev Bras Ortop (Sao Paulo) 2019;54(3):275–81.

5. Kohls-Gatzoulis J, Angel JC, Singh D, et al. Tibialis posterior dysfunction: a common and treatable cause of adult acquired flatfoot. BMJ 2004;329(7478): 1328–33.

6. Merrill RK, Ferrandino RM, Hoffman R, et al. Identifying risk factors for 30-day readmissions after triple arthrodesis surgery. J Foot Ankle Surg 2019;58(1):109–13.

7. Soukup DS, MacMahon A, Burket JC, et al. Effect of obesity on clinical and radiographic outcomes following reconstruction of stage ii adult acquired flatfoot deformity. Foot Ankle Int 2016;37(3):245–54.

8. Conti MS, Jones MT, Savenkov O, et al. Outcomes of reconstruction of the stage ii adult-acquired flatfoot deformity in older patients. Foot Ankle Int 2018;39(9): 1019–27.

9. Yang Z., Liu F., Cui L., et al., Adult rigid flatfoot: triple arthrodesis and osteotomy, Medicine (Baltimore), 99 (7), 2020, 1–5.

10. Hoke M. An operation for stabilizing paralytic feet. Am J Orthop Surg 1921;3: 494–507.

11. Knupp M, Stufkens SA, Hintermann B. Triple arthrodesis. Foot Ankle Clin 2011; 16(1):61–7.

12. Burrus MT, Werner BC, Carr JB, et al. Increased failure rate of modified double arthrodesis compared with triple arthrodesis for rigid pes planovalgus. J Foot Ankle Surg 2016;55(6):1169–74.

13. Fadle AA, El-Adly W, Attia AK, et al. Double versus triple arthrodesis for adult-acquired flatfoot deformity due to stage III posterior tibial tendon insufficiency: a prospective comparative study of two cohorts. Int Orthop 2021;45(9):2219–29.

14. Schuh R, Salzberger F, Wanivenhaus AH, et al. Kinematic changes in patients with double arthrodesis of the hindfoot for realignment of planovalgus deformity. J Orthop Res 2013;31(4):517–24.

15. Jia X, Qiang M, Chen Y, et al. The influence of selective arthrodesis on three-dimensional range of motion of hindfoot joint: a cadaveric study. Clin Biomech (Bristol, Avon) 2019;69:9–15.

16. Astion DJ, Deland JT, Otis JC, et al. Motion of the hindfoot after simulated arthrodesis. J Bone Joint Surg Am 1997;79(2):241–6.

17. Wülker N, Stukenborg C, Savory KM, et al. Hindfoot motion after isolated and combined arthrodeses: measurements in anatomic specimens. Foot Ankle Int 2000;21(11):921–7.

18. Berlet GC, Hyer CF, Scott RT, et al. Medial double arthrodesis with lateral column sparing and arthrodiastasis: a radiographic and medical record review. J Foot Ankle Surg 2015;54(3):441–4.

19. Roche AJ, Calder JD. Lateral column lengthening osteotomies. Foot Ankle Clin 2012;17(2):259–70.

20. Suckel A, Muller O, Herberts T, et al. Talonavicular arthrodesis or triple arthrodesis: peak pressure in the adjacent joints measured in 8 cadaver specimens. Acta Orthop 2007;78(5):592–7.

21. Smith NC, Beaman D, Rozbruch SR, et al. Evidence-based indications for distraction ankle arthroplasty. Foot Ankle Int 2012;33(8):632–6.

22. Sammarco VJ, Magur EG, Sammarco GJ, et al. Arthrodesis of the subtalar and talonavicular joints for correction of symptomatic hindfoot malalignment. Foot Ankle Int 2006;27(9):661–6.

23. Evans D. Calcaneo-valgus deformity. J Bone Joint Surg Br 1975;57(3):270–8.

24. Conti SF, Wong YS. Osteolysis of structural autograft after calcaneocuboid distraction arthrodesis for stage II posterior tibial tendon dysfunction. Foot Ankle Int 2002;23(6):521–9.

25. Thomas RL, Wells BC, Garrison RL, et al. Preliminary results comparing two methods of lateral column lengthening. Foot Ankle Int 2001;22(2):107–19.

26. Li HM, Lui TH. Correction of severe flatfoot deformity by 3-portal arthroscopic triple arthrodesis. Arthrosc Tech 2019;9(1):e103–9.

27. Coetzee JC, Hansen ST. Surgical management of severe deformity resulting from posterior tibial tendon dysfunction. Foot Ankle Int 2001;22(12):944–9.

28. Seybold JD, Coetzee JC. Primary triple arthrodesis for management of rigid flatfoot deformity. JBJS Essent Surg Tech 2016;6(3):e29.

29. Ryerson E. Arthrodesing operations on the feet. J Bone Joint Surg Am 1923;5: 453–71.

30. Ohly NE, Cowie JG, Breusch SJ. Triple arthrodesis of the foot with allograft through a lateral incision in planovalgus deformity. Foot Ankle Surg 2016;22(2): 114–9.

31. Hyer CF, Galli MM, Scott RT, et al. Ankle valgus after hindfoot arthrodesis: a radiographic and chart comparison of the medial double and triple arthrodeses. J Foot Ankle Surg 2014;53(1):55–8.

32. Phisitkul P, Haugsdal J, Vaseenon T, et al. Vascular disruption of the talus: comparison of two approaches for triple arthrodesis. Foot Ankle Int 2013;34(4): 568–74.

33. Mulfinger GL, Trueta J. The blood supply of the talus. J Bone Joint Surg Br 1970; 52(1):160–7.

34. MacDonald A, Anderson M, Soin S, et al. Single medial vs 2-incision approach for double hindfoot arthrodesis: is there a difference in joint preparation? Foot Ankle Int 2021;42(8):1068–73.

35. Bono JV, Jacobs RL. Triple arthrodesis through a single lateral approach: a cadaveric experiment. Foot Ankle 1992;13(7):408–12.

36. Jeng CL, Vora AM, Myerson MS. The medial approach to triple arthrodesis. indications and technique for management of rigid valgus deformities in high-risk patients. Foot Ankle Clin 2005;10(3):515–21.

37. Jackson WF, Tryfonidis M, Cooke PH, et al. Arthrodesis of the hindfoot for valgus deformity. an entirely medial approach. J Bone Joint Surg Br 2007;89(7):925–7.

38. Weinraub GM, Schuberth JM, Lee M, et al. Isolated medial incisional approach to subtalar and talonavicular arthrodesis. J Foot Ankle Surg 2010;49(4):326–30.

39. Brilhault J. Single medial approach to modified double arthrodesis in rigid flatfoot with lateral deficient skin. Foot Ankle Int 2009;30(1):21–6.

40. So E, Reb CW, Larson DR, et al. Medial double arthrodesis: technique guide and tips. J Foot Ankle Surg 2018;57(2):364–9.

41. Miniaci-Coxhead SL, Weisenthal B, Ketz JP, et al. Incidence and radiographic predictors of valgus tibiotalar tilt after hindfoot fusion. Foot Ankle Int 2017; 38(5):519–25.

42. Lui TH. Arthroscopic triple arthrodesis in management of chronic flatfoot deformity. Arthrosc Tech 2017;6(3):e871–7.

43. Lui TH. New technique of arthroscopic triple arthrodesis. Arthroscopy 2006;22(4): 464.e1–5.

44. Walter R, Parsons S, Winson I. Arthroscopic subtalar, double, and triple fusion. Foot Ankle Clin 2016;21(3):681–93.

45. Talarico LM, Vito GR. Triple arthrodesis using external ring fixation and arched-wire compression: an evaluation of 87 patients. J Am Podiatr Med Assoc 2004; 94(1):12–21.

46. Schipper ON, Ford SE, Moody PW, et al. Radiographic results of nitinol compression staples for hindfoot and midfoot arthrodeses. Foot Ankle Int 2018;39(2): 172–9.

47. Meyer MS, Alvarez BE, Njus GO, et al. Triple arthrodesis: a biomechanical evaluation of screw versus staple fixation. Foot Ankle Int 1996;17(12):764–7.

48. Payette CR, Sage RA, Gonzalez JV, et al. Triple arthrodesis stabilization: a quantitative analysis of screw versus staple fixation in fresh cadaveric matched-pair specimens. J Foot Ankle Surg 1998;37(6):472–80.

49. Chuckpaiwong B, Easley ME, Glisson RR. Screw placement in subtalar arthrodesis: a biomechanical study. Foot Ankle Int 2009;30(2):133–41.

50. Saragaglia D, Giunta JC, Gaillot J, et al. Subtalar arthrodesis using a single compression screw: a comparison of results between anterograde and retrograde screwing. Eur J Orthop Surg Traumatol 2021. https://doi.org/10.1007/s00590-021-03141-7.

51. DeCarbo WT, Berlet GC, Hyer CF, et al. Single-screw fixation for subtalar joint fusion does not increase nonunion rate. Foot Ankle Spec 2010;3(4):164–6.

52. Haskell A, Pfeiff C, Mann R. Subtalar joint arthrodesis using a single lag screw. Foot Ankle Int 2004;25(11):774–7.

53. McGlamry MC, Robitaille MF. Analysis of screw pullout strength: a function of screw orientation in subtalar joint arthrodesis. J Foot Ankle Surg 2004;43(5): 277–84.

54. Boffeli TJ, Reinking RR. A 2-screw fixation technique for subtalar joint fusion: a retrospective case series introducing a novel 2-screw fixation construct with operative pearls. J Foot Ankle Surg 2012;51(6):734–8.

55. Vacketta V.G., Jones J.M., Philp F.H., et al., Radiographic outcomes of talonavicular joint arthrodesis with varying fixation techniques in stage iii adult acquired flatfoot reconstruction, J Foot Ankle Surg, 61 (5), 2022, 969–974.

56. Kiesau CD, Larose CR, Glisson RR, et al. Talonavicular joint fixation using augmenting naviculocalcaneal screw in modified double hindfoot arthrodesis. Foot Ankle Int 2011;32(3):244–9.

57. Milshteyn MA, Dwyer M, Andrecovich C, et al. Comparison of two fixation methods for arthrodesis of the calcaneocuboid joint: a biomechanical study. Foot Ankle Int 2015;36(1):98–102.

58. Kann JN, Parks BG, Schon LC. Biomechanical evaluation of two different screw positions for fusion of the calcaneocuboid joint. Foot Ankle Int 1999;20(1):33–6.

Ankle Joint Salvage for Rigid Flatfoot Deformity

Kshitij Manchanda, MD*, George Tye Liu, DPM, Matthew J. Johnson, DPM, Michael D. Van Pelt, DPM, Katherine M. Raspovic, DPM, Dane K. Wukich, MD

KEYWORDS

- Ankle arthritis • Ankle arthroplasty • Ankle replacement • Flatfoot • Valgus ankle

KEY POINTS

- The cause of flatfoot is multifactorial and poorly understood.
- Medial ankle instability is the primary cause of ankle valgus, which occurs in long-standing flatfoot deformities.
- Treatment of this instability can vary from nonoperative to operative intervention.
- Operative interventions may require ligamentous reconstruction, osteotomies, arthrodesis, arthroplasty, or a combination of these procedures.
- In cases of severe hindfoot deformity with ankle arthritis, staging the procedure to correct the hindfoot deformity first is preferred before performing total ankle replacement (TAR). As TAR technology and long-term survivorship improves, more patients would benefit and favor an ankle replacement over an ankle arthrodesis.

INTRODUCTION

Medial ankle instability with a rigid flatfoot deformity is a complex clinical condition of which management strategies continue to evolve. The flatfoot deformity requires correction to alleviate the pronation stress that results in attenuation of the superficial and deep deltoid ligament complex and subsequent ankle valgus deformity. As we further our understanding of the anatomy and the biomechanics of this deformity, we know that this is an interaction that involves multiple joints and soft tissue elements in different planes. This allows us to explore different treatment options and individualize management strategies for each patient.

PATHOANATOMY AND BIOMECHANICS

Flatfoot pathologic condition is complex and multifactorial. The posterior tibial tendon is the initial soft tissue structure, which contributes to the posterior tibial tendon dysfunction, also referred to as adult acquired flat foot deformity.

Department of Orthopaedic Surgery, University of Texas Southwestern Medical Center, 1801 Inwood Road, Dallas, TX 75390-8883, USA
* Corresponding author.
E-mail address: kshitij.manchanda@utsouthwestern.edu

Clin Podiatr Med Surg 40 (2023) 333–340
https://doi.org/10.1016/j.cpm.2022.11.010
0891-8422/23/Published by Elsevier Inc.

podiatric.theclinics.com

The posterior tibial tendon functions as the primary supinator of the foot, locking the transverse tarsal joint to create a rigid lever during toe off and terminal midstance of gait. Posterior tibial tendon dysfunction can be caused by degenerative disease, inflammatory conditions, or metabolic diseases. Histopathologic examination has shown disruption in collagen bundle structure, disruption of the posterior tibial tendon through mucinous degeneration, and fibroblast hypercellularity which may predispose it to injury under physiologic loads.[1] Once the posterior tibial tendon becomes insufficient, the antagonist pull of the peroneus brevis muscle overpowers the posterior tibial muscle inhibiting the locking mechanism of the transverse tarsal joint. The vertical ground reactive force of push-off therefore transfers from the metatarsal head to the talar head.[2] Over time, the spring (calcaneonavicular) ligament complex becomes attenuated leading to arch collapse, forefoot abduction, and hindfoot valgus. The pronation stress transmits to the ankle, which eventually causes superficial and deep deltoid ligament attenuation and resultant ankle valgus deformity.

The spring and deltoid ligament has been studied in its contribution to flatfoot formation. Previous anatomic studies have shown the confluence of the superficial deltoid with the spring ligament complex, suggesting that both structures provide stability to the medial tibiotalar and talonavicular joints, and therefore, subsequent injury or degenerative changes to these tissues can lead to progressive medial column instability and flatfoot deformity.[3]

Changes in osseous anatomy focus on the triple joint complex particularly around peritalar subluxation.[4] With the advent of weight-bearing computed tomography scan, we are now able to identify the associated position of the joints of the triple complex with foot deformity. For example, congenital pes planovalgus deformity, resulting in increased valgus orientation of the subtalar joint could be predisposing a subset of patients to develop a symptomatic flatfoot deformity that can involve the ankle, hindfoot, and midfoot.[5]

ETIOLOGY/EPIDEMIOLOGY

The prevalence of rigid flatfoot within the general population is largely unknown. Many people with flatfeet are asymptomatic and flexible, never seeking medical consultation.[6]

Symptomatic flatfoot deformity may present with medial hindfoot pain over the posterior tibial tendon, deep plantar pain over the spring ligament, or lateral subfibular impingement in more advanced stages. Additionally, some adult patients can present with symptomatic, rigid flatfoot deformities secondary to tarsal coalition as well.[7]

The cause of flatfoot is still an evolving concept. Historically, posterior tibialis tendon dysfunction has been seen as the major inciting factor; however, there are other static structures such as the deltoid ligament, spring ligament, and plantar fascia that maintain arch height in the foot.[8]

CLASSIFICATION AND STAGING

There are 6 staging classifications, with the first being published by Johnson and Strom in 1989.[9] Their classification relied on defining the deformity by 3 stages, which was then subsequently updated to add a stage IV by Myerson. Stage I is defined by tenosynovitis of the posterior tibial tendon with no deformity and normal hindfoot inversion with single-limb heel rise. Stage II begins to highlight increased degeneration and weakness to the posterior tibial tendon with a flexible and reducible pes planovalgus deformity. With stage III, the deformity is more fixed and irreducible. Stage IV additionally demonstrates valgus deformity of the ankle.

Subsequent classification systems are modifications of this classification. Overall, the consensus of these classifications reflects a difference between rigid and flexible flatfoot deformities, which guides treatment. In 2019, the Progressive Collapsing Foot Deformity (PCFD) classification was devised, which relies on both anatomy and function. After defining whether the deformity is rigid or flexible, 5 deformity patterns are analyzed: hindfoot valgus, midfoot/forefoot abduction, forefoot varus/medial column instability, peritalar subluxation, and ankle instability. This classification system provides a systematic method to classify/diagnose the deformity and develop a treatment plan. Additionally, the classification scheme highlights that PCFD is progressive, and that it does not always progress from once stage to another, at times it skips steps between the deformity patterns (**Table 1**).[10]

ANKLE INSTABILITY IN FLATFOOT

When discussing ankle instability in flatfoot patients, it is important to understand the role of the deltoid ligament. The superficial component comprises the tibionavicular ligament, tibiospring ligament, tibiocalcaneal ligament (strongest portion), and the posterior superior tibiotalar ligament. This ligamentous complex is the primary restraint to tibiotalar valgus angulation. The deep component comprises the posterior and anterior tibiotalar ligaments and inserts on the talus to control axial rotation of the talus. The deep components prevent lateral displacement of the talus and acts as a restraint against external rotation. The deltoid ligament is often overlooked on examination of the patient with posterior tibial tendon dysfunction.[8,11]

When examining the original Johnson and Strom flatfoot classification system along with the Myerson modification, stage IV deformities (or Class E in PCFD classification) are generally associated with valgus tilting of the talus. Concomitantly, the hindfoot may be in stage II or III depending on the flexibility. Stage IV disease is rare and has been reported to affect 2.3% of the total population.[12] Stage IV has 2 substages: A

Table 1
Progressive collapsing foot deformity classification—consensus classification in 2020

Progressive Collapsing Foot Deformity Classification 2020		
Stages of deformity		
Stage I	Flexible	
Stage II	Rigid	
Types of deformity (Classes—isolated or combined)		
Class A	Hindfoot valgus deformity	Hindfoot valgus alignment Increased hindfoot moment arm, hindfoot alignment angle, foot and ankle offset
Class B	Midfoot/forefoot abduction deformity	Decreased talar head coverage Increased talonavicular coverage angle, presence of sinus tarsi impingement
Class C	Forefoot varus deformity/ medial column instability	Increased talus-first metatarsal angle Plantar gapping first tarsometatarsal joint/naviculocuneiform joints Clinical forefoot varus
Class D	Peritalar subluxation/ dislocation	Significant subtalar joint subluxation/ subfibular impingement
Class E	Ankle instability	Valgus tilting of the ankle joint

(flexible without significant arthritis) and B (rigid hindfoot arthritis or significant tibiotalar arthritis).

Medial ankle instability can be difficult to detect, therefore thorough clinical and diagnostic evaluation is important to determine the stage of the deformity and therefore plan for treatment. Clinically, patients will have pain along their medial gutter and increased hindfoot valgus with weight-bearing. Weight-bearing foot and ankle radiographs are important to visualize the deformities in detail and to perform comparisons bilaterally. Assessing ankle valgus can be best seen on an anterior-posterior ankle radiograph, which can show the morphology of the tibiotalar joint and reveal any medial collateral ligament laxity or talar angular displacement (**Fig. 1**).[7] Advanced imaging such as MRI can be helpful in identifying discontinuity of the deltoid ligament when radiographs do not show joint malalignment. Whether this is clinically useful in dictating surgical treatment and affecting long-term patient outcomes is largely unknown.[13]

NONOPERATIVE TREATMENT

Before surgical intervention, nonoperative modalities should be considered for all patients. Although these options do not correct the deformity, nonoperative options may provide significant pain relief and potentially delay the need for surgical treatment. These options include articulating and nonarticulating ankle foot orthoses with a medial hindfoot postincorporated to relieve the valgus ankle collapse.

OPERATIVE TREATMENT

When nonoperative treatment fails to provide relief, surgery is considered. Managing ankle valgus with posterior tibial tendon dysfunction is determined by the reducibility of the ankle deformity and presence of ankle arthritis. If reducible with limited arthritic changes, then either deltoid ligament reconstruction, supramalleolar (or malleolar repositioning) osteotomies, or a combination of these may be considered. With severe

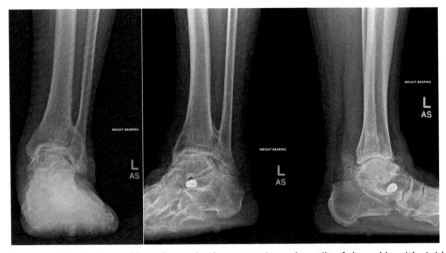

Fig. 1. Weight-bearing ankle radiographs demonstrating valgus tilt of the ankle with rigid hindfoot arthritis.

ankle arthritic changes, either pantalar fusion or hindfoot realignment arthrodesis with a total ankle replacement (TAR) has been a more reliable option.[7]

Addressing the flatfoot deformity, the first goal is to achieve a plantigrade and well-aligned foot; otherwise, ankle reconstructive attempts may fail if there is any residual deformity.[14] For the flexible hindfoot deformity, calcaneal osteotomy and flexor digitorum longus tendon transfers can be performed but as our discussion centers around rigid deformities, this indicates arthritic changes and nonreducible contractures of the hindfoot joints. Therefore, realignment hindfoot arthrodesis should be considered in these situations.[8]

Regarding the ankle, there are various options for treatment of the valgus instability. Joint-sparing options are commonly preferred because they place less stress on neighboring joints. If the goal is retaining ankle range of motion, then the deformity needs to be carefully assessed. Brunner and colleagues[15] defined treatment guidelines based on the location of the deformity (supramalleolar, intra-articular, inframalleolar). If the deformity is supramalleolar, then a supramalleolar osteotomy should be performed. However, when the deformity is through the joint, then the amount of tibiotalar height loss, the valgus tilt, and the amount of medial clear space widening are factors considered in ankle reconstruction. Reconstruction of the deltoid ligament should be considered when there is more than 10° of valgus tilt or 5 mm of medial clear space because this indicates deltoid insufficiency. If the medial dome of the talus is below the medial malleolus, this is also an indication that the deltoid ligament is insufficient. A TAR should only be performed in a congruent joint; otherwise, this can lead to edge loading and eccentric polyethylene wear. TAR failure rates are higher in patients with more than 10° of angular deformities.[15] If there is any concern about the deltoid ligament intraoperatively, this should be appropriately reconstructed to avoid catastrophic failure. Based on our experience, increasing the polyethylene thickness also can improve sagittal instability but this can constrain the entire joint and affect range of motion. However, no studies have been published to quantify the improvement seen with increasing polyethylene thickness.

Therefore, before performing a TAR, the foot should be plantigrade and well aligned and the reconstruction of the medial collateral ankle ligaments may be required. Staging the surgery is often preferred in these cases, especially when performing adjunctive fusions because of the concern for avascular necrosis of the talus. If the rigid flatfoot deformity cannot be aligned through realignment arthrodesis of the foot, and the ankle cannot be balanced with medial collateral ligament reconstruction, TAR is contraindicated.[16,17] Residual flatfoot deformities may cause abnormal ankle kinematics and tibiotalar contact pressures. Cadaveric studies have shown that flatfoot deformity shifts the tibiotalar contact area laterally and decreases the contact area by 35%.[18] Residual hindfoot valgus places excessive stress to the medial ankle, leading to failure of the deltoid and further progression of ankle instability.

The question remains whether patients with significant valgus deformities do well with ankle replacements. Demetracopolous and colleagues[19] demonstrated improved patient-reported outcomes in patients who underwent total ankle arthroplasty with moderate-to-severe valgus deformities. Overall, correction was maintained and outcomes improved at 1 year and final follow-up. The outcomes from this study indicate that ankle replacement can be a viable alternative to ankle arthrodesis in patients with severe ankle valgus deformities with a well-aligned foot.[19]

Similarly, Queen and colleagues[20] reported an observational study on 103 patients who underwent TAR. They reported improved coronal alignment was associated with improved outcome scores and walking speeds. Analyses between subgroups (ie, preoperative neutral vs valgus versus varus alignments) did not demonstrate any significant differences, indicating that patients with the severest of deformities can also do well as long as the ankle and foot deformities are appropriately corrected.[20]

Mobile-bearing TARs have been popular outside the United States.[21–24] A South Korean study with a minimum 4-year follow-up of a mobile-bearing design reported similar outcomes in patients with varus or valgus ankle malalignment up to 20° when compared with the preoperative neutral alignment patients. There were neither reported differences with complications nor functional outcome scores between the groups indicating that correction of the coronal plane deformity associated with successful outcomes.[21] A subsequent study reported that the survival probability and patient reported outcomes scores were similar between the severe (20°–35°) and moderate (5°–15°) deformity corrected groups.[22]

Isolated ankle realignment arthrodesis may be performed in cases of ankle valgus with arthritis. Similar to ankle replacement, the concomitant foot deformity should be plantigrade and must be well aligned to achieve satisfactory results.[23] Therefore, combination of ankle and hindfoot realignment arthrodesis such as provided by a tibiotalocalcaneal or pantalar fusion can help establish a plantigrade foot. Although the patients generally improve compared with their preoperative baselines, one limitation of a pantalar fusion is creating significant stiffness to the lower extremity sometimes requiring the use of orthopedic shoes and accommodative insoles to address residual pain. These patients may also have increased energy expenditures and decreased function versus patients with preserved joints.[24] Ankle-sparing procedures should be considered in patients with congruent joints or ankle joint where congruity can be restored through realignment/reconstructive procedures. Gait studies have demonstrated significant improvements for ankle arthroplasty patients in various parameters including sagittal dorsiflexion, higher walking velocities due to increases in stride length and cadence, and more normalized gait cycle. Even the stiffest of ankles have maintained improvements in range of motion at intermediate and long-term follow-ups.[25,26]

Anecdotally, patients with stage IV flatfoot deformities with relatively preserved ankle range of motion prefer maintaining ankle range of motion. Patients without preserved range of motion seem to accept arthrodesis and a stiff ankle better than patients with preserved ankle range of motion.

Overall, patients' perceptions also affect their outcomes. Insight into patients with an ankle arthrodesis or replacement is viewed with advantages and disadvantages. Although patients with ankle arthrodesis reported that the ankle seemed stable and strong, it also seemed stiffer.[27] With the improvement in ankle replacement technology and advent of many soft tissue reconstruction procedures, more studies are being published suggesting that TAR has equivalent or better outcomes than ankle arthrodesis in patients with ankle valgus pathologic condition with concomitant advanced PCFD.

SUMMARY

In summary, ankle valgus may develop in long-standing rigid flatfoot deformities. Nonoperative treatment consists of bracing/orthoses. Surgical interventions include ligamentous reconstruction, osteotomies, arthrodesis, arthroplasty, or a combination of these procedures, depending on clinical and imaging characteristics of the deformity. In some cases of ankle arthritis, when significant hindfoot deformity is present, staged correction of the hindfoot deformity first before total ankle arthroplasty is recommended. As TAR technology and survivorship continues to advance, more patients may benefit from total ankle arthroplasty compared with ankle arthrodesis.

CLINICS CARE POINTS

- Ankle valgus with long-standing rigid flatfoot deformities can be operatively treated with ligamentous reconstructions, osteotomies, arthrodesis, arthroplasty, or a combination of these procedures.

- These deformities can either be operatively treated with pantalar arthrodesis or hindfoot realignment arthrodesis with a TAR.

- It is vital to have a plantigrade foot before performing a total ankle arthroplasty to avoid eccentric or "edge loading" of the polyethylene.

- In patients with significant hindfoot deformity and ankle arthritis, a staged correction allows for improved outcomes and management postoperatively.

- Gait studies demonstrate significant improvements for ankle arthroplasty patients in various parameters during gait. Therefore, range of motion should be preserved whenever possible.

DISCLOSURE

Dr G.T. Liu is a consultant for Orthofix and Gramercy Extremity Orthopedics and has equity interest with Gramercy Extremity Orthopedics. Dr K.M. Raspovic is a consultant for Orthofix. Dr D.K. Wukich is a consultant for Orthofix, Wright Medical Technologies, Stryker, and Arthrex. He receives royalties from Arthrex.

REFERENCES

1. Mosier SM, Pomeroy G, Manoli A 2nd. Pathoanatomy and etiology of posterior tibial tendon dysfunction. Clin Orthop Relat Res 1999;365:12–22.
2. Deland JT, de Asla RJ, Sung IH, et al. Posterior Tibial Tendon Insufficiency: which ligaments are involved? Foot Ankle Int 2005;26(6):427–35.
3. Campbell KJ, Michalski MP, Wilson KJ, et al. The ligament anatomy of the deltoid complex of the ankle: a qualitative and quantitative anatomical study. J Bone Joint Surg Am 2014;96(8):e62.
4. Anathakrisnan D, Ching R, Tencer A, et al. Subluxation of the talocalcaneal joint in adults who have symptomatic flatfoot. J Bone Joint Surg Am 1999;81(8):1147–54.
5. Apostle KL, Coleman NW, Sangeorzan BJ. Subtalar joint axis in patients with symptomatic peritalar subluxation compared to normal controls. Foot Ankle Int 2014;35(11):1153–8.
6. Godoy-Santos AL, Schmidt EL, Chaparro F. What are the updates on epidemiology of progressive collapsing foot deformity? Foot Ankle Clin N Am 2021;26:407–15.
7. Toullec E. Adult flatfoot. Orthop Traumatol Surg Res 2015;101(1Suppl):S11–7.
8. Plaass C, Louwerens JW, Claassen L, et al. Treatment concepts for pes valgo planus with concomitant changes of the ankle joint : tibiotalocalcaneal arthrodesis, total ankle replacement and joint-preserving surgery. Orthopade 2020;49(11):991–9. English. Erratum in: Orthopade. 20Mar;50(3):244.
9. Johnson KA, Strom DE. Tibialis posterior tendon dysfunction. Clin Orthop Relat Res 1989;239:196–206.
10. Myerson MS, Thordarson DB, Johnson JE, et al. Classification and nomenclature: progressive collapsing foot deformity. Foot Ankle Int 2020;41(10):1271–6.
11. Cain JD, Dalmau-Pastor M. Anatomy of the deltoid-spring ligament complex. Foot Ankle Clin N Am 2021;26:237–47.

12. Bluman E, Myerson M. Stage IV posterior tibial tendon rupture. Foot Ankle Clin 2007;12:341–62.
13. Chhabra A, Soldatos T, Chalian M, et al. 3-Tesla magnetic resonance imaging evaluation of posterior tibial tendon dysfunction with relevance to clinical staging. J Foot Ankle Surg 2011;50(3):320–8.
14. Smith JT, Bluman EM. Update on stage IV acquired adult flatfoot disorder when the deltoid ligament becomes dysfunctional. Foot Ankle Clin 2012;17:351–60.
15. Brunner S, Knupp M, Hintermann B. Total ankle replacement for the valgus unstable osteoarthritic ankle. Tech Foot Ankle Surg 2010;9:165–74.
16. Schuberth JM, Christensen JC, Seidenstricker CL. Total ankle replacement with severe valgus deformity: technique and surgical strategy. J Foot Ankle Surg 2017;56:618–27.
17. Dodd A, Daniels TR. Total ankle replacement in the presence of talar varus or valgus deformities. Foot Ankle Clin 2017;22(2):277–300.
18. Friedman MA, Draganich LF, Toolan B, et al. The effects of adult acquired flatfoot deformity on tibiotalar joint characteristics. Foot Ankle Int 2001;22(3):241–6.
19. Demetracopoulos CA, Cody EA, Adams SB Jr, et al. Outcomes of total ankle arthroplasty in moderate and severe valgus deformity. Foot Ankle Spec 2019;12(3): 238–45.
20. Queen RM, Adams SB Jr, Viens NA, et al. Differences in outcomes following total ankle replacement in patients with neutral alignment compared with tibiotalar joint malalignment. J Bone Joint Surg Am 2013;95(21):1927–34.
21. Lee GW, Wang SH, Lee KB. Comparison of intermediate to long-term outcomes of total ankle arthroplasty in ankles with preoperative varus, valgus, and neutral alignment. J Bone Joint Surg Am 2018;100(10):835–42.
22. Lee GW, Lee KB. Outcomes of total ankle arthroplasty in ankles with >20° of coronal plane deformity. J Bone Joint Surg Am 2019;101(24):2203–11.
23. Colin F, Zwicky L, Barg A, et al. Peritalar instability after tibiotalarfusion for valgus unstable ankle in stage IV adult acquired flatfoot deformity. Foot Ankle Int 2013; 34:1677–82.
24. Tenenbaum S, Coleman SC, Brodsky JW. Improvement in gait following combined ankle and subtalar arthrodesis. J Bone Joint Surg Am 2014;96:1863–9.
25. Flavin R, Coleman SC, Tenenbaum S, et al. Comparison of gait after total ankle arthroplasty and ankle arthrodesis. Foot Ankle Int 2013;34(1):1340–8.
26. Brodsky JW, Jaffe D, Pao A, et al. Long-term functional results of total ankle arthroplasty in stiff ankles. Foot Ankle Int 2021;42(5):527–35.
27. Conlin C, Khan RM, Wilson I, et al. Living with both a total ankle replacement and an ankle fusion: a qualitative study from the patients' perspective. Foot Ankle Int 2021;42(9):1153–61.

Approach to the Ankle in Adult Acquired Flatfoot Deformity

Mark J. Capuzzi, DPM, AACFAS[a,b,]*, Jason R. Miller, DPM[a,b,c],
Tymoteusz Siwy, DPM[d,1]

KEYWORDS

- Flatfoot • Adult acquired flatfoot deformity • Posterior tibial tendon dysfunction
- Ankle valgus • Rearfoot valgus • Progressive collapsing flatfoot • Ankle arthroplasty
- Tibiotalocalcaneal arthrodesis

KEY POINTS

- Understand the biomechanics of the ankle in relationship to flatfoot deformity.
- Understand the purpose of operative versus non operative treatment as it relates to the ankle in progressive flatfoot deformity.
- Propose a treatment algorithm specific to ankle pathomechanics with progressive collapsing flatfoot deformity.

INTRODUCTION

Flatfoot deformity is commonly encountered by foot and ankle specialists. It can also be known or diagnosed concurrently with adult acquired flatfoot deformity (AAFD), pes planovalgus, flexible valgus deformity, hypermobile flatfoot, posterior tibial tendon dysfunction (PTTD), or peroneal spastic flatfoot, depending on its cause. Recently, the orthopedic community has made attempts to standardize the nomenclature by using progressive collapsing flatfoot deformity.[1,2] The deformity is not invariably symptomatic, with fewer than 15% of adults with flatfoot becoming symptomatic. Among the symptomatic patients, most are middle-aged female, with history of obesity, diabetes, hypertension, equinus, or participation in high-impact sports.[1–5]

[a] Pennsylvania Intensive Lower Extremity Fellowship Program, Malvern, PA, USA; [b] Foot & Ankle Surgery, Premier Orthopedics/Pennsylvania Orthopaedic Center, 266 West Lancaster Avenue, Suite 200, Malvern, PA 19355, USA; [c] Surgical Residency Program, Department of Surgery, Tower Health/Phoenixville Hospital Podiatric Medicine, PMSR/RRA, Temple University, Phoenixville, PA, USA; [d] Surgical Residency Program, Tower Health/Phoenixville Hospital Podiatric Medicine and Surgery Residency, PMSR/RRA, Phoenixville, PA, USA
[1] Present address: 245 South Cedar Street, APT C212, Spring City, PA 19475.
* Corresponding author.
E-mail address: Mjc5527@gmail.com

Clin Podiatr Med Surg 40 (2023) 341–349
https://doi.org/10.1016/j.cpm.2022.11.011
podiatric.theclinics.com

Clinically, patients present with complaints of pain in the medial longitudinal arch, posteromedial ankle, and occasionally subfibular area and over the sinus tarsi. Pain can be aggravated by prolonged standing and weightbearing activity. In addition, patients may note flattening of their medial longitudinal arch on weight-bearing. With more advanced deformity, edema above the medial ankle may be present and the deformity may become irreducible.[1,3,6]

On physical examination, tenderness can frequently be elicited along the course of the posterior tibial (PT) tendon and sometimes in the lateral heel, distal to the lateral malleolus. Isolated manual muscle testing of the PT muscle should be performed to assess for insufficiency; this may also elicit pain in a patient with symptomatic PTTD. On weight-bearing, a collapse of the medial longitudinal arch may be noted along with "too many toes sign." The hindfoot may be in valgus with the forefoot compensating in varus, or the forefoot may be in varus with the subtalar joint compensating by resting in valgus.[1,3,6] The patient may have difficulty performing a single heel rise with pain, and as the deformity progresses, a lack of varus rotation of the heel may be noted with the heel rise, and eventually the patient may be unable to perform a single heel rise.[1–3,5–7]

The most common associated pathology of progressive collapsing flatfoot deformity is PTTD. The PT tendon is an important foot pronator and a major stabilizer of the medial longitudinal arch. PTTD is a progressive dysfunction starting as inflammation, progressing through intrasubstance tears, and potentially complete rupture of the tendon. A hypovascular zone is present in the retromalleolar portion of the tendon, with supply vessels entering the tendon approximately 2 cm distal and 4.5 cm proximal to the medial malleolus. Hypovascularity as well as mechanical stress in the retromalleolar space are cited as a potential cause of failure of the tendon.[8,9] In addition, as the PT tendon fails, the spring ligament has been implicated, as it is the main static medial arch stabilizer and it fails in 74% to 92% of patients with PT tendon tears.[1,5]

AAFD has a multifactorial pathology. As procedures and technologies have evolved, there are a variety of new techniques surgeons can explore for deformity correction of the AAFD. As surgeons, it is critical to have a concise algorithm for correcting deformity. The aim of the present paper is to present the most current diagnostic and therapeutic approaches to treatment of the ankle in end-stage AAFD.

Staging of Adult Acquired Flatfoot Deformity

Historically, classification systems and clinical stages of certain pathologies related to the foot and ankle can provide not only diagnostic clues but aid in treatment algorithms. Johnson and Strom first described 3 stages of PTTD in 1989 and a fourth was later added by Myerson. The aim of this paper is to focus on the ankle as it pertains to the AAFD; however, it is critical to make the young surgeon aware of these clinical stages. Staging a patient is an excellent starting point for a treatment algorithm in the treatment of the adult acquired flatfoot.

Stage I is characterized by pain and swelling of the medial aspect of the foot and ankle. The length of the tendon is normal, and tendinitis may be associated with mild degeneration. Mild weakness and minimum deformity are present. In stage II, the tendon is torn, the limb is weak, and the patient is unable to stand on tiptoe on the affected side. Secondary deformity is present as the midfoot pronates and the forefoot abducts at the transverse tarsal joint. The subtalar joint, however, remains flexible. In stage III, degeneration of the tendons present, the deformity is more severe, and the hindfoot is rigid. Stage IV, proposed by Myerson, is characterized by valgus angulation of the talus and early degeneration of the ankle joint.[10,11] A more comprehensive classification system that addresses the diversity of the AAFD was presented by Bluman and Myerson in 2007. This revised classification offers a more detailed discussion of each clinical stage and provides treatment options for the complex problem of AAFD (**Table 1**).[12]

Stage IV disease occurs in the setting of long-standing PTT rupture and is most often associated with deltoid ligament insufficiency leading to a valgus ankle deformity.[12] Stage 4 PTT insufficiency implies the additional attrition and elongation of the deep deltoid ligament, enabling valgus tilting of the talus within the ankle mortise.[13] Ankle valgus results from the lateral tilt of the talus as a consequence of the deltoid ligament failure. Stage IVA is characterized by hindfoot valgus with flexible ankle valgus without significant ankle arthritis. Stage IVB refers to hindfoot valgus with rigid ankle valgus or flexible ankle valgus with significant arthritis.[4] Deltoid ligament complex insufficiency is a fundamental pathologic component of stage IV AAFD. Failure of the deltoid ligament allows the talus to tilt into valgus within the ankle mortise. If left untreated, ankle joint biomechanics are altered and may lead to debilitating tibiotalar arthritis.[14]

Clinical Presentation with Diagnostic Evaluation of the Ankle Adult Acquired Flatfoot Deformity

Physical examination is critical in the diagnosis and management of the AAFD. All evaluations should be done on B/L lower extremities, and should involve an NWB examination, followed by a WB examination, and lastly a gait evaluation to ascertain any pathology proximally to the hindfoot and ankle (**Fig. 1**). As the deformity progresses to Stage III and beyond, which is the focus of this discussion, the classic medial-sided pain along the course of the PTT is usually absent, as the tendon is likely ruptured as the valgus ankle progresses. It is important to rule out any acute tarsal tunnel symptoms with the long-standing valgus tilt of the hindfoot and ankle.[15,16] Hindfoot valgus should be noted and can be roughly estimated by visualizing through a goniometer to the patient's hindfoot. A history of associated ankle weakness and swelling is common. Patients frequently present with a multitude of failed braces, orthotics, and shoes. As the ankle valgus becomes more of a fixed deformity, forces are transferred to the fibula, where a stress fracture is possible, termed Johnson stage V disease.[17]

Eliciting pain at the lateral aspect of the hindfoot suggests subfibular impingement, manifesting as pain within the sinus tarsi. Patients with stages III or IV may also experience pain on palpation of arthritic joints across the hindfoot and ankle. The most likely findings in these later stages are a pronounced valgus deformity of the hindfoot with deltoid insufficiency and an inability to heel rise. Pain and callus pattern at the talonavicular joint are often present secondary to dorsolateral peritalar subluxation, causing prominence at the medial plantar midfoot.[12] Chronic eccentric loading of the ankle joint in valgus creates lateral compartment arthritic wear patterns, and the examiner will elicit pain within the lateral ankle gutter. The lateral ankle pain with which a patient in stage 3 would present is now only partially subfibular impingement and more directly related to ankle arthritis.[18]

Radiographic Evaluation

Radiographic evaluation of the flatfoot deformity begins with at least an anteroposterior (AP) and lateral foot radiographs. On the AP view, one can assess talonavicular coverage angle. It is the angle formed by the intersection of lines formed at the articular surface of the talar head and the proximal articular surface of the navicular. This angle is ideally 0°, and normal value falls less than 7°. Calcaneocuboid angle is obtained by drawing a tangent line on the lateral aspect of the cuboid and the lateral edge of the calcaneus. Normal CC angle falls in 0° to 5° range. Angles greater than

Table 1
Simplified Bluman-Myerson classification of the adult acquired flatfoot deformity

Stage	Deformity	Disease Progression	Treatment
I	None	PTT tendinosis or tenosynovitis Functional tendon	Conservative treatment initially tenosynovectomy
II			
IIA	Flexible moderate deformity (<40% of the talar head uncovered)	Tendinosis or a low-to-moderate tear of the PTT Laxity of the spring ligament	Orthoses Tendon transfer Medializing calcaneal osteotomy Subtalar arthroereisis Medial column stabilizing procedure
IIB	Flexible severe deformity (>40% of the talar head uncovered or subtalar impingement)	High-grade tear of PTT Incompetent spring ligament Sinus tarsi syndrome	Consider adding lateral column lengthening reconstruction
III	Rigid (inflexible) deformity	Subtalar osteoarthrosis Lateral hindfoot impingement	Subtalar arthrodesis or triple arthrodesis Consider adding medial ray procedure for plantar flexion of the first metatarsal
IV			
IVA	Flexible tibiotalar valgus	Deltoid ligament abnormality	Flatfoot reconstruction and deltoid ligament reconstruction
IVB	Rigid tibiotalar valgus	Tibiotalar osteoarthrosis	Consider adding tibiotalar fusion or ankle arthroplasty

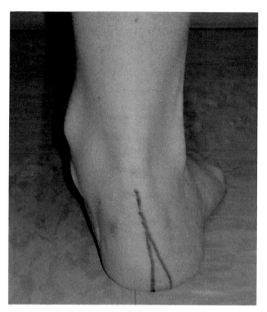

Fig. 1. Hindfoot evaluation of adult acquired flatfoot deformity.

5° are seen in planus type feet. Talocalcaneal angle, also known as kite's angle, is also commonly evaluated. This angle is formed from the intersection of lines drawn along the lateral border of the calcaneus and the line bisecting the talar head and neck. Normal values are between 25° and 40°, with an angle greater than 40° indicating rearfoot valgus and angles less than 25° indicating rearfoot varus. The alignment of the talar axis and the first metatarsal shaft may also be evaluated by drawing a line along the long axis of the first metatarsal and the talus. In a rectus foot, the axis of the talus and the axis of the first metatarsal will be parallel or nearly parallel. If the talar line is angled medial to the axis of the first metatarsal shaft axis, it can indicate a planus deformity.[1,5,9]

Meary angle can be measured on lateral radiographs. It is the angle between the long axes of the talus and the first metatarsal. The normal value of Meary angle is 0° to 4°. Mild disease is manifested by angles between 4° and 15°. Moderate disease has a Meary angle between 15° and 30°. Severe disease is denoted by an angle greater than 30°. Calcaneal inclination angle is likewise linked with pes planus deformity. This angle is measured by intersecting lines drawn parallel to weight-bearing surface and the plantar calcaneal border. An angle greater than 30° denotes a cavus foot, whereas an ankle less than 18° indicates a planus foot. Cyma line is a lazy S-shaped line drawn across the TN and CC joints on AP and lateral projections. In a rectus foot, the line should be continuous. Anterior displacement of the TN joint is attributed to pes planus.[1,5,6]

More advanced disease warrants a set of ankle radiographs. As the deformity progresses into stage IV, increasing valgus angulation of the talus in the tibiotalar joint can be observed. Subtalar arthritis may be observed on lateral projection in stage III and above. Stage IVB may also show signs of degeneration at the ankle joint, with considerable narrowing at the medial tibiotalar joint.[1,5,9]

Other imaging modalities are used to assess adult acquired flatfoot. MRI can visualize the PT tendon and any deficiencies thereof. The deltoid and spring ligament pathology may also be detected with the use of an MRI. Computed tomography scans are useful in detecting bony coalitions and arthritic changes at the tibiotalar, subtalar, and talonavicular joints present in more advanced disease.[5]

Surgical Approaches to the Ankle in End-Stage Adult Acquired Flatfoot Deformity

Joint sparing procedures typically consist of deltoid ligament reconstruction with distal realignment. Attempts to address the ankle pathology with isolated reconstruction of the deltoid ligament without realignment of the foot deformity will result in recurrence. Deland and colleagues described reconstruction of the deltoid ligament by passing a peroneus longus tendon graft through a bone tunnel in the talus from lateral to medial and then through a second tunnel from the tip of the medial malleolus to the lateral tibia. Five patients underwent bony correction of the foot deformity followed by deltoid reconstruction with the peroneal tendon graft. At 2-year follow-up all patients had maintained correction of the talar tilt.[19] Minimally invasive deltoid ligament repair in conjunction with triple arthrodesis has been proposed by Jeng and colleagues as a new treatment option that allows for preservation of ankle motion in patients diagnosed with stage IV disease who have less than 10° of valgus tibiotalar.[20] In a cadaveric study by Haddad, a novel technique of correcting the superficial and deep deltoid ligament was proposed in 2010. The anterior tibial tendon was harvested, and tunnels were created in the distal tibia at the deltoid origin and at the talus (deep) and calcaneus (superficial) deltoid insertions. Then placed through torque measurements, this reconstruction technique under low torque was able to restore eversion and external rotation stability to the talus, which was statistically similar to the intact deltoid ligament.[21] Bluman and Myerson described their technique with a forked hamstring allograft for reconstruction of both the superficial and deep deltoid complex. This minimally invasive technique involves reconstruction with a 20 cm hamstring allograft split longitudinally, creating 2 limbs for insertion into the talus and calcaneus.[22]

In the more rigid deformities, the surgical options become a bit more limited to larger fusions. The authors typically reserve the pantalar arthrodesis for patients with rigid ankle valgus, and/or an ankle valgus of greater than 15°, and the patients who would not be candidates to total ankle replacement (diabetic, morbid obesity, heavy tobacco usage). Although a reliable treatment option for stage IV AAFD, the pantalar arthrodesis comes with several complications, including nonunion, which is most common, infection, hardware failure, wound healing, and loss of limb.[23,24] Patients should be aware of these complications, and it should be relayed by the surgeon that loss of limb is a realistic complication with any pantalar arthrodesis. The pantalar arthrodesis remains a salvage procedure in our hands and is limited to the aforementioned comorbid patients.

Tibiotalocalcaneal arthrodesis remains a better option than the pantalar arthrodesis. Tibiotalocalcaneal arthrodesis is another option in the treatment algorithm. Although very rare that the talonavicular joint and calcaneocuboid joint would be spared in the long-standing stage IV AAFD, it remains a viable option in treating the valgus ankle. Patients with tibiotalocalcaneal arthrodesis tend to be improved but will have continued pain and limited activity.[17,25]

As previously stated, most valgus ankles will have severe deformity in the hindfoot best treated by realignment and arthrodesis of the talonavicular and subtalar joints. In these cases, in which extensive surgical dissection around the medial and lateral sides of the talus is needed for hindfoot correction, it is not wise to perform total ankle replacement at the same time. Bohay and Anderson propose that patients with a relatively flexible flatfoot may be treated with conventional osteotomy or triple arthrodesis, an additional total ankle arthroplasty in a staged procedure.[17] Although some procedures such as medializing calcaneal osteotomy and subtalar fusions can be performed

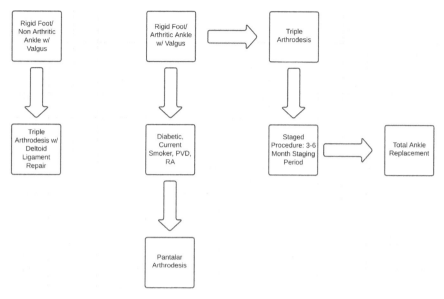

Fig. 2. PAILEF AAFD stage IV surgical treatment algorithm.

at the time of prosthesis implantation, it has been recommended that more extensive procedures (eg, triple arthrodesis) be done at least 3 months before total ankle arthroplasty.[26,27] Total ankle replacement is a viable option for preservation of the motion at the ankle joint. Bonin and colleagues recommend a 45-day staging time frame before the total ankle arthroplasty following triple arthrodesis. In their series, 2-stage total ankle replacements were done in 18 patients and found no morbidity was associated with 2-stage total ankle replacement. They did, however, note a lower American Orthopedic Foot and Ankle Society score in patients who underwent both procedures (total ankle arthroplasty and triple arthrodesis). They attribute this to the loss of subtalar joint motion.[28]

Vulcano and colleagues, in 2013, offered a broad treatment algorithm for the treatment of stage III and IV AAFD.[4] At the authors' institution they follow a similar surgical treatment plan when addressing the ankle in end-stage AAFD. They propose the following treatment algorithm for the first time in literature to be shared for review and use in practice (**Fig 2**). They offer this treatment algorithm for the young surgeons to have in their arsenal when faced with the difficulty of surgical planning for the end-stage AAFD.

SUMMARY

AAFD or progressive collapsing flatfoot deformity is a deformity of not just the foot but rather a progressive deformity that affects the subtalar joint and the ankle in later stages. Although conservative treatment may be effective in alleviating the symptoms of disease in earlier stages, more aggressive approaches are required for definitive treatment and treatment of end stage of the disease. Flexible deformities may be amenable to joint sparing intervention.[19–21] Rigid deformities and deformities with more than 10° talar valgus are more likely to require joint destructive procedures. These procedures are patient specific and range from an isolated subtalar joint arthrodesis through triple, pantalar, and tibiotalocalcaneal arthrodesis. Appropriate patients may also be eligible for a staged approach, with total ankle arthroplasty as the final procedure. We propose a treatment algorithm designed with stage IV patients in mind, and hope this helps the young surgeon in preoperative planning of this complicated deformity.

CLINICS CARE POINTS

- Flatfood deformity is progressive in nature to the foot & ankle.
- As the deformity becomes more rigid, the ankle pathology requires evaluation and treatment.
- Non operative and operative treatments are appropriate management of rigid stage IV flatfoot deformity.

DISCLOSURE

The authors declare that they have no known competing financial interests or personal relationships that could have seemed to influence the work reported in this paper.

REFERENCES

1. Jackson JB 3rd, Pacana MJ, Gonzalez TA. Adult acquired flatfoot deformity. J Am Acad Orthop Surg 2022;30(1):e6–16. PMID: 34932505.
2. Myerson MS, Thordarson DB, Johnson JE, et al. Classification and nomenclature: progressive collapsing foot deformity. Foot Ankle Int 2020;41(10):1271–6. Epub 2020 Aug 28. PMID: 32856474.
3. Deland JT. Adult-acquired flatfoot deformity. J Am Acad Orthop Surg 2008;16(7): 399–406. PMID: 18611997.
4. Vulcano E, Deland JT, Ellis SJ. Approach and treatment of the adult acquired flatfoot deformity. Curr Rev Musculoskelet Med 2013;6(4):294–303. PMID: 23765382; PMCID: PMC4094099.
5. Flores DV, Mejía Gómez C, Fernández Hernando M, et al. Adult acquired flatfoot deformity: anatomy, biomechanics, staging, and imaging findings. Radiographics 2019;39(5):1437–60.
6. Institute TP, Southerland , Alder . McGlamry's comprehensive textbook of foot and ankle surgery, 2. Philadelphia: Wolters Kluwer Health; 2012. Chapter 44.
7. Ling SK, Lui TH. Posterior tibial tendon dysfunction: an overview. Open Orthop J 2017;11:714–23. PMID: 28979585; PMCID: PMC5620404.
8. Manske MC, McKeon KE, Johnson JE, et al. Arterial anatomy of the tibialis posterior tendon. Foot Ankle Int 2015;36(4):436–43. Epub 2014 Nov 19. PMID: 25411117.
9. Toullec E. Adult flatfoot. Orthop Traumatol Surg Res 2015;101(1 Suppl):S11–7. Epub 2015 Jan 13. PMID: 25595429.
10. Johnson KA, Strom DE. Tibialis posterior tendon dysfunction. Clin Orthop Relat Res 1989;239:196–206.
11. Myerson MS. Adult acquired flatfoot deformity: treatment of dysfunction of the posterior tibial tendon. InstrCourse Lect 1997;46:393–405.
12. Bluman EM, Title CI, Myerson MS. Posterior tibial tendon rupture: a refined classification system. Foot Ankle Clin 2007;12(2):233–49.
13. Kelly Ir, Nunley JA. Treatment of stage 4 adult acquired flatfoot. Foot Ankle Clin 2001;6(1):167–78.

14. Smith JT, Bluman EM. Update on stage IV acquired adult flatfoot disorder. Foot Ankle Clin 2012;17(2):351–60.
15. Daniels TR, Lau JT, Hearn TC. The effects of foot position and load on tibial nervetension. Foot Ankle Int 1988;19(2):73–8.
16. Francis H, March L, Terenty T, et al. Benign joint hypermobility with neuropathy:-documentation and mechanism of tarsal tunnel syndrome. J Rheumatol 1987; 14(3):577–8.
17. Bohay DR, Anderson JG. Stage iv posterior tibial tendon insufficiency: the tilted ankle. Foot Ankle Clin 2003;8:619–36.
18. Coughlin MJ, Mann RA, Saltzman CL. Surgery of the foot and ankle. 8th Edition. Philadelphia: Mosby-Elsevier; 2007.
19. Deland JT, de Asla RJ, Segal A. Reconstruction of the chronically failed deltoidligament: a new technique. Foot Ankle Int 2004;25:795–9.
20. Jeng CL, Bluman EM, Myerson MS. Minimally invasive deltoid ligament reconstruction for stage IV flatfoot deformity. Foot Ankle Int 2011;32(1):21–30.
21. Haddad SL, Dedhia S, Ren Y, et al. Deltoid Ligament Reconstruction: A Novel Tech Biomechanical Anal Foot Ankle Int 2010;31(7):639–51.
22. Bluman EM, Myerson MS. Stage IV posterior tibial tendon rupture. Foot Ankle Clin 2007;12:341–62.
23. Barrett GR, Meyer LC, Bray EW, et al. Pantalar arthrodesis: a long-term follow-up. Foot & Ankle 1981;1(5):279–83.
24. Acosta R, Ushiba J, Cracchiolo A. The results of a primary and staged pantalar arthrodesis and tibiotalocalcaneal arthrodesis in adult patients. Foot Ankle Int 2000;21(3):182–94.
25. Papa JA, Myerson MS. Pantalar and tibiotalocalcaneal arthrodesis for post-traumatic osteo-arthritis of the ankle and hindfoot. J Bone Joint Surg 1992; 74A(7):1042–9.
26. Stamatis ED, Myerson MS. How to avoid specific complications of total ankle replacement. Foot Ankle Clin 2002;7(4):765–89.
27. Bluman EM, Chiodo CP. Valgus ankle deformity and arthritis. Foot Ankle Clin 2008;13(3):443–70.
28. Bonnin M, Judet T, Colombier JA, et al. Midterm results of the salto total ankle prosthesis. Clin Orthopaedics Relat Res 2004;424:6–18.

Surgical Considerations for Revision Flatfoot Reconstruction

Overcorrection/Undercorrection

Sandeep Patel, DPM[a,b,]*, John M. Schuberth, DPM[b,c], Matthew Cobb, DPM[d], Craig E. Krcal Jr, DPM[b,1]

KEYWORDS

- Flatfoot reconstruction • Revision flatfoot reconstruction
- Adult acquired flatfoot reconstruction • Flatfoot surgery outcomes

KEY POINTS

- Over- and undercorrection of flatfoot deformities account for poor outcomes and are often multiplanar.
- Long-standing deformities are more difficult to correct due to bony adaptation.
- Revision should be performed at the apex of deformity, and osteotomies should be made through prior arthrodesis sites if necessary.
- Achieving a plantigrade foot results in improved function, pain relief, and shoe wear

INTRODUCTION

Flatfoot deformities are a common pathologic condition treated by the foot and ankle surgeons. Patients will often present with an array of symptoms including poster tibial tendinitis, midfoot pain, lateral column discomfort, and ultimately developing degenerative changes in the midfoot and hindfoot. When patients fail conservative management, they often undergo surgical intervention. Over the years, numerous surgical approaches have been recommended to address the chronic symptoms associated with flatfoot deformities. These procedures have ranged from simple soft-tissue reconstruction and rebalancing, to corrective osteotomies and selective arthrodesis. The success of the surgery often depends on choosing the appropriate procedure

[a] Diablo Service Area, Kaiser Permanente, 1425 South Main Street, Walnut Creek, CA 94596, USA; [b] Kaiser San Francisco Bay Area, Foot and Ankle Residency Program, Oakland, CA, USA; [c] Department of Orthopedic Surgery, 450 6th Avenue, San Francisco, CA 94115, USA; [d] 8080 Academy Road NE Suite C, Albuquerque, NM 87111, USA

[1] Present address: 3600 Broadway, Oakland, CA 94611, USA.

* Corresponding author.

E-mail address: sbpatel21@gmail.com

Clin Podiatr Med Surg 40 (2023) 351–364

https://doi.org/10.1016/j.cpm.2022.11.005

0891-8422/23/© 2022 Elsevier Inc. All rights reserved.

given the patient's unique deformity, appreciating the apex of the deformity, and considering other patient factors such as age, bone stock, underlying comorbidities, and weight.

Poor outcomes are often a result of early complications such as infection and wound complications, nonunion, and malunion. The focus of this review is to discuss the management of failed flatfoot reconstruction, specifically over- and undercorrection of the flatfoot deformity. There are several factors that may contribute to these outcomes including failure to recognize initial deformity, intraoperative malposition, or poor fixation that would allow the recurrence of the deformity. In addition, surgeons are often limited by their training and limit their procedure selection to their familiarity. A failure to recognize any underlying neuromuscular disorder or tendon imbalance that may also result in progressive deformity.

BACKGROUND

Flatfoot deformity encompasses a large spectrum of foot and ankle pathology with varying degrees of severity and treatment needs. This pathology is present in the pediatric population with etiologies ranging from asymptomatic, idiopathic, and reducible to symptomatic and rigid due to congenital calcaneovalgus, vertical talus, or tarsal coalitions.[1–4] It is possible to encounter these pathologies as a sequalae of untreated congenital pathology in adults; however, we are most often confronted with the management of symptomatic flatfoot as seen with a progressive adult-acquired flatfoot deformity (AAFD).

In 1989 Johnson and Strom published a landmark article describing the progression of adult-acquired flatfoot that is still used in assessing tibialis posterior tendon pathology and flatfoot progression. Their original classification described the progression of AAFD in four stages ranging from tendinous pathology and symptomatology to rigid deformity with ankle involvement.[5] This classification is prognostic in nature with conservative therapy in the form of physical therapy, bracing, and prevention of progression of deformity as the first line of treatment in patients with reducible deformities.[6–8] On the contrary, recalcitrant pain, worsening of deformity, or initial presentation with end-stage rigid deformity may ultimately warrant surgical management of the symptomatic flatfoot deformity.

Generally speaking, younger patients and patients with reducible deformities who fail conservative therapy are offered joint sparring procedures such as posterior tibialis (PT) tendon debridement and retubularization with advancement, flexor digitorum longus (FDL) transfer, medial displacement calcaneal osteotomy (MDCO), Evans osteotomy or a combination of the above. In contrast, patients with more progressive deformities and arthritis are typically offered arthrodesis to correct larger deformities and to resolve arthritic joint pain in the form of tarsometatarsal (TMT), naviculocuneiform (NC) talonavicular (TN), subtalar joint (STJ), calcaneocuboid (CC) arthrodesis or a combination of the above or with triple arthrodesis and or soft-tissue balancing procedures.[9]

It has proven to be difficult to compare radiographic or clinical outcomes of flatfoot reconstruction given the diverse procedure selection which is ultimately guided by surgeon preference and patient symptoms and architecture. Conti and colleagues[10] set out to formally assess the optimal position of the heel following reconstruction of stage II AAFD with MDCO and they found mild radiographic varus following osteotomy fixation to be predictive of the greatest improvement in clinical outcomes following hindfoot reconstruction measured with FAOS scores.

Day and colleagues[4] looked at 71 patients with flexible flatfoot and divided this population into two groups based on age. Rearfoot arthrodesis was excluded from results and treatment ranged from Evans osteotomy, to FDL transfer, first TMTJ fusion, and PT tendon repair based on the discretion of a fellowship-trained attending surgeon. Using the Patient Reported Outcome Measurement Information Systems (PROMIS) they found both subsets of patients to significantly benefit from AAFD reconstruction, but younger patients maintained greater physical function with comparable radiographic correction and less frequent indication for tendon transfers, arthrodesis or other additional corrective surgeries as seen at the 2-year mark with 36.4% minor reoperation rate in the younger group including hardware removal. Conversely, they found a 38.9% reoperation rate, major and minor, in the older group suggesting younger patients with AAFD may have a lower risk of major reoperation rate than older patients when considering joint sparing procedures.

Adult-acquired flatfoot in its later stages can be particularly debilitating and the need for more extensive correction in the form of rearfoot arthrodesis may be necessary for symptom management and deformity correction. Functional outcomes were looked at by Beischer and colleagues[11] after triple or double arthrodesis were evaluated in a small patient population which revealed excellent or good outcomes as they relate to AOFAS scores following rearfoot double or triple arthrodesis for the treatment of AAFD or posttraumatic arthritis in %76 of their patients. Rohm and colleagues[12] published mid to long term outcomes of hindfoot fusions with rigid flatfoot deformity in 96 consecutive modified triple arthrodesis with a single medial approach. AOFAS scores with a mean follow-up time of 4.9 years revealed 66% very good or good patient satisfaction, and mean AOFAS score at the final follow-up of 67 points, and a mean FAOS pain subscale of 72.6. Of note, patients with "bad" satisfaction scores were 16% and these patients were noted to have a greater progression of flatfoot deformity including tibiotalar tilt and a higher rate of substantial comorbidities that may indicate a poorer prognosis for more advanced AAFD flatfoot reconstruction.

Ultimately, the aim of flatfoot reconstruction is to remove planovalgus forces throughout the foot and ankle to alleviate strain on soft-tissue and to eliminate arthritic progression or symptomatology by balancing tendinous and osseous architecture. Outcomes depend on a case-by-case basis with the most predictable outcomes coming from proper patient workup, correct procedure choice, execution, and proper reduction of the deformities.

When outcomes of flatfoot reconstruction do not meet patient expectations and the patient remains symptomatic or displeased, a detailed understanding of anatomy, biomechanics and treatment options must be thoroughly assessed before revision consideration. Outcomes resulting in persistent symptomatology range from nonunion to malunion as seen with undercorrection and overcorrection. A plethora of reasons, both host and iatrogenic can play a role in nonunion including but not limited to atrophic nonunion, poor preparation of an arthrodesis site, ill-conceived fixation constructs. When assessing symptoms without concerns for nonunion; however, over or undercorrection are typically the root cause. Common residual symptoms following flatfoot reconstruction indicating overcorrection include—lateral column stiffness, overloading of the lateral column, proximal or distal joint stiffness or pain from the area of correction, peroneal tendonitis or spasm, sub-metatarsal head callosity, sesamoiditis or stress fractures.[13] Symptoms indicating undercorrection may include persistent preoperative pain, PT tendonitis, and plantar fasciitis.[14]

Maenpaa and colleagues[15] reported 307 triple arthrodesis in patients with rheumatoid arthritis. Of the patients that had a poor outcome, 66% were a result of malunion. Of those, a valgus malalignment was more common than a varus malalignment. The authors also commented that varus malalignment, or overcorrections, are less forgiving and poorly tolerated by patients. This is our experience as well. Slight undercorrection or residual valgus can often be accommodated with orthotic therapy, shoe modifications, and bracing; conversely, it is difficult to accommodate the over-corrected flatfoot reconstruction with a varus rearfoot.

The literature on the management of failed flatfoot reconstruction is sparse. Most of the literature is based on small series and established algorithms for identifying the level of deformity and stepwise approach to correction.[16,17] Haddad and colleagues[16] reviewed the clinical and radiographic outcomes of revision surgery for failed triple arthrodesis. They proposed a surgical algorithm to determine procedures to correct the deformity based on alignment and symptoms. The study included a total of 29 feet that presented with some form of deformity, 10 of which were multiplanar. After following their protocol, their patient cohort was found to have a marked improvement in AOFAS scores, and overall alignment based on clinical and radiographic assessment. Despite having a 14% rate of major complications, all patients stated they would have the surgery again.

Toolan reported on revision of failed triple arthrodesis using an opening–closing wedge osteotomy of the midfoot in five patients.[17] He performed a multiplanar osteotomy removing a truncated wedge medially and inserting it laterally. The intention was to correct the deformity while avoiding an excessive shortening of the foot. He noted improvement in the radiographic parameters of the AP and lateral talo-first metatarsal angle and valgus talar tilt which correlated with an improvement in AOFAS scores, less pain, improved function, and improved footwear.

PATIENT EVALUATION

The preoperative evaluation is multifaceted. In addition to identifying the symptomatic presentation, it is also important to obtain a thorough past medical history. Specifically, underlying neuromuscular disorders should be identified and assessed to ensure the over or under-correction was not the direct result of poor execution of prior procedures, but rather the result of a progressive deformity. The overwhelming majority of neuromuscular imbalances are occult and one is not likely to benefit from the operative notes of the past but the radiographs are far more revealing to uncover covert imbalances. The patient may also provide a history that the foot was doing well early on after the index surgery, but over time, it has deformed.

In addition, obtaining prior surgical reports to determine which procedures were performed will aid in surgical planning. It is important to understand the rationale behind the procedures that were initially performed as well as any tendon transfers that may have taken place, as this may dictate or limit soft-tissue reconstruction during revision attempts.

A thorough physical examination should be performed to determine the precise location of pain, areas of callus formation indicating focal pressure overload and osseous prominences, and the level of rigidity (**Fig. 1**). A dynamic examination to account for the muscle imbalance, function, and contracture is also a necessary component in surgical planning.

Finally, obtaining appropriate imaging is paramount. Standard radiographs should initially be obtained in each case. It is also important to obtain ankle images to assure there is no acquired deformity as well as calcaneal axial views to appreciate calcaneal alignment in relation to the long axis of the tibia (**Fig. 2**). It may also be beneficial to obtain images of the contralateral foot as a reference, especially if the contralateral foot is asymptomatic and relatively well aligned. As mentioned before, CT scans can provide additional information regarding the presence of a nonunion as well as providing three-dimensional images of the overall alignment (**Fig. 3**).

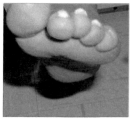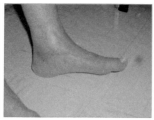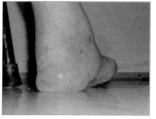

Fig. 1. Non-weightbearing and weightbearing clinic examination of the patient show a rigid forefoot varus malalignment.

CONSIDERATIONS

There are numerous factors that need to be considered when evaluating the failed flat-foot reconstruction. When patients present with persistent symptoms, it is important to rule out nonunion. This is readily assessed by evaluating plain film radiographs for persistent patency across osteotomies or fusion sites, fractured hardware, or loss of correction from the initial radiographs. Furthermore, advanced imaging in the form of computed tomography (CT) scans, must be considered when ruling out a nonunion or assessing malalignment. Not only does it provide valuable information regarding osseous bridging or consolidation at arthrodesis or osteotomy sites, it provides a three-dimensional characterization of the alignment of the foot. The vast majority of the time, the malalignment is related to osseous malposition or failure to perform the appropriate index procedure.

Finally, the presence of muscular imbalance should not be overlooked. This is especially important in failed flatfoot surgery that may have originally had an adequate

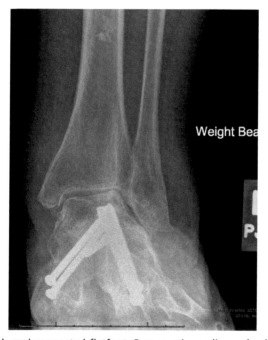

Weight Bea

Fig. 2. Patient with undercorrected flatfoot. Preoperative radiographs show valgus tilt of the ankle joint.

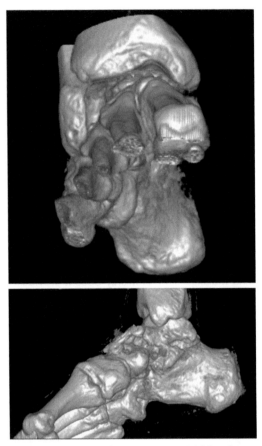

Fig. 3. Three-dimensional CT rendering demonstrating rigid forefoot varus deformity.

correction. Tendon imbalance, whether it is the result of an underlying neuromuscular disorder or tendon attrition, can result in progressive deformity in joints proximal and distal to previous arthrodesis sites. In addition, any untreated equinus contracture can result in a continued deforming force on the hindfoot and midfoot.

As with any reconstructive surgery, outcomes and patient satisfaction are often correlated with appropriate alignment. Numerous radiographic parameters are described in the literature to assess the alignment of the foot in both the AP and lateral projections.[18–21] However, correcting the talo-first metatarsal angle on both the AP and lateral projection has been shown to have a high correlation with patient satisfaction.[17] Furthermore, these are relatively simple parameters to assess with intraoperative imaging in a simulated weightbearing film. However, it should be stressed that no imaging study can determine the torsional deformation of the foot. The radiographs only show one-dimensional correction and normalizing these angles does to necessarily assure a plantigrade foot.

SURGICAL TECHNIQUES

Regardless of the type of failed flatfoot reconstruction, the concepts for revising the under- and overcorrected flatfoot reconstruction remain the same. The ultimate goal is to achieve a plantigrade foot, improve pain and function, and allow for use of over-the-counter shoe wear. As mentioned before, the level of deformity in the various planes must be identified individually with a plan for corrective procedures to address calcaneal alignment, midfoot abduction/adduction, and forefoot varus/valgus. Different surgical techniques and algorithms have been described to guide surgical management.[16,17] The authors agree with these general principles with an emphasis on identifying the apices of deformity as the ideal area of correction. In addition, any acquired degenerative changes in proximal and distal joints should be considered to assure long-term pain relief.

Undercorrected

These deformities are often a result of truly corrected flatfeet or progressive deformity overtime. As previously mentioned, these can often be multiplanar and require a thorough evaluation to ensure a plantigrade foot when considering revision. The primary deformities include persistent hindfoot valgus, compensated forefoot varus/supinatus, and abduction of the midfoot, and potentially a rocker bottom deformity. These deformities along with any soft-tissue constraints need to be considered and approached in a stepwise manner intraoperatively.

Hindfoot valgus

Valgus alignment of the hindfoot can be addressed in one of two ways. Patients with a previous STJ arthrodesis at the index procedure may benefit from a medializing calcaneal osteotomy.[22] This options is only practical for a mild valgus deformity, An oblique incision is placed through standard approach on the lateral heel just posterior to the anticipated location of the sural nerve. Following the preferred method of osteotomy, the calcaneal tuberosity should be translated approximately 1 to 1.5 cm medially with every attempt to realign the heel underneath the tibial axis. In most cases however, if the STJ has been fused and is still in valgus, you have to cut through the fusion mass as close to the STJ axis as possible from a medial approach; moving the heel will not alter the vertical vector through the ankle, still causing a valgus thrust.

If a patient underwent prior calcaneal osteotomy with recurrent valgus deformity, consideration should be made in performing an STJ arthrodesis as there is always a potential for some level of STJ instability. This may result in the persistent valgus alignment of the heel which can be addressed by STJ arthrodesis. This procedure has been shown to provide multiplanar correction.[23]

Forefoot varus

Once the heel is aligned, there will often be a residual deformity in the midfoot, in particular a varus deformity. The goal is to restore the alignment of the medial column such that the first ray will achieve purchase upon weight bearing. There are various techniques to address this pathology, including arthrodesis of one or multiple joints in the medial column depending on the level of the fault. If all the joints are well aligned, consideration can be made for a cotton osteotomy.[24]

However, if a prior medial column arthrodesis was performed and was malaligned, the recommendation would be to revise the fusion site. A prior malaligned triple arthrodesis is an excellent example. The revision is performed through a medial and lateral-based incision to adequately protect the soft-tissue envelope. Upon subperiosteal dissection, malleable retractors are placed both dorsally and plantarly to allow safe passage of the oscillating saw for the revision osteotomy. The use of k-wires is recommended to template the placement of the osteotomy. Multiple views under intraoperative fluoroscopy should be used to verify the placement of the pin in the osteotomy. Typically, the osteotomy is made from media to lateral which allows rotation of the forefoot upon the hindfoot to realign the medial column, thus recreating the tripod effect of the foot (**Fig. 4**).

Forefoot abduction and rockerbottom deformity

These deformities can be corrected through a similar approach for the management of a complicated varus deformity with the addition of a wedge resection. For isolated abduction deformity, a medial-based biplanar wedge can be removed. Again, the utilization of pins to aid in performing the osteotomy can be beneficial. A proximal pin can be inserted from medial to lateral, perpendicular to the axis of the hindfoot. A second pin is then inserted from medial to lateral perpendicular to the long axis of the second metatarsal to converge the pins on the lateral aspect of the foot. This will allow for adequate removal of the medial-based wedge to reduce the deformity. Alternatively, the size of the medial-based wedge can be predetermined with the utilization of preoperative radiographs. Current software available to surgeons alongside electronic images has simplified operative planning and should be used.

In the setting of a concomitant rockerbottom deformity, a truncated wedge is removed with a plantar medial-based wedge. Erring on the side of removing less bone is recommended as residual deformity can be fine-tuned with reciprocal planning.

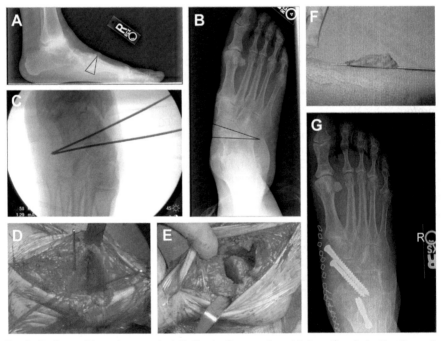

Fig. 4. Patient with undercorrected flatfoot after previous triple arthrodesis. Continues to have a varus and abduction deformity of the forefoot with possible nonunion of the TN joint. (*A, B*) Preoperative template. (*C–F*) Demonstration of intraoperative guidewire placement to remove a truncated wedge. The wires are placed under fluoroscopic guidance. Figure Y6 shows the successful removal of the wedge. (*G*) Postoperative radiographs show improved alignment of the forefoot abduction deformity. The lines in B are proposed osteotomy based off of imaging software. The lines in C represnt the insertion of steinman pins to template the osteotomy

Overcorrected

This is the more unforgiving type of malalignment. These often occur more as a result of hindfoot arthrodesis or excessive graft utilization during an Evan's osteotomy. Furthermore, excessive Plantar flexion of the medial column will result in increased load to the first ray. The patient will essentially present with symptoms similar to a cavus foot type. As with the under-corrected flatfoot, each level of deformity needs to be assessed to restore a plantigrade foot type.

Hindfoot varus

The approach to the deformity is based on the patient's underlying symptoms and prior procedures. If the symptoms are related to hindfoot instability or peroneal tendon pathology, the various deformity can be addressed with the calcaneal osteotomy. This osteotomy can be performed with a lateral-based wedge along with lateral translation if needed. However, if the patient underwent prior STJ arthrodesis, with lateral column symptoms, a simple osteotomy may not be sufficient. In this scenario, a more aggressive osteotomy with a lateral based wedge through the prior arthrodesis site may be necessary. The osteotomy should be as close to the joint axis as possible for optimal correction.

Forefoot valgus

In essence, this is a plantarflexed first ray. Depending on the level of prior corrective procedure, a dorsiflexory osteotomy can be made at the apex of deformity. Alternatively, if the patient had a prior triple arthrodesis that is healed in varus malalignment, an osteotomy is made through the prior TN and CC joints. Similar to addressing a forefoot varus deformity, a medial and lateral incision is placed with subperiosteal dissection. A wire is used to orient the direction of the osteotomy. The bone cut is made across the prior arthrodesis site and the foot can then be rotated back into neutral alignment, perpendicular to the hindfoot.

Forefoot adduction

Adduction of the forefoot is often restored with hindfoot correction. However, if there is residual adduction of the forefoot after addressing the hindfoot varus, a lateral-based wedge can be removed from the midfoot. This is essentially the opposite of correcting an abduction deformity. Other factors to consider are the previous surgeries performed. If the patient had an Evans osteotomy with excessive graft size, consideration for shortening the lateral column is an option. The most effective and predictable way to perform this would be through a CC joint arthrodesis (**Fig. 5**). It can be technically

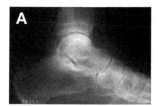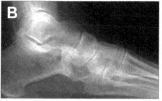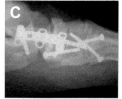

Fig. 5. (*A*) Patient with flatfoot symptoms, primarily in the medial column. (*B*) Patient underwent a lateral column lengthening procedure and overcorrected the hindfoot while neglecting the medial column fault. This is an example of inappropriate procedure choice possibly based on surgeon's training and lack of appreciating the nuances of flatfoot reconstruction. Notice the overcorrection of the TN joint. (*C*) Revision of the surgery included a CC joint fusion with wedge resection and medial column arthrodesis. Note more anatomic alignment of the TN joint on the lateral projection.

demanding to get good opposition of the arthrodesis surfaces and consideration for releasing the talo-navicular joint and medial soft-tissue contractures needs to be considered.

Soft-tissue Considerations

Tightness of the gastrocnemius–soleus complex and Achilles tendon are common findings in flatfoot deformity. Although this is commonly addressed at the index procedure, recurrent contracture is common and should be addressed during the revision surgery. Overlengthening is less common and can result in a calcaneus gait. If encountered, reconstruction and tendon transfer may be necessary.

Other tendons to evaluate are the FDL and peroneal tendons. If the tendon was transferred initially resulting in overcorrection, the tendon should be released or lengthened. If the tendon was not initially transferred, and the correction is deficient, then use of the tendon to serve as a dynamic balancing force can be a useful augmentation during the revision procedure. This is more pertinent in cases where hindfoot arthrodesis procedures can be avoided to obtain the correction.

Case examples
Case I. Patient presented with initial symptoms consistent with AAFD **Fig. 6**.

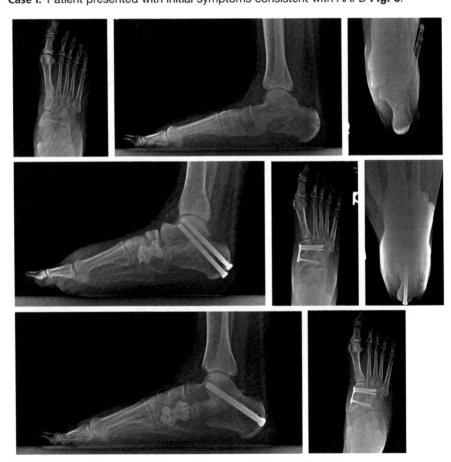

Fig. 6. Patient presented with initial symptoms consistent with AAFD.

During the index procedure, the patient underwent STJ arthrodesis, NC joint arthrodesis, and gastrocnemius lengthening. In this case, the STJ was overcorrected.

The revision considerations for this patient included a lateralizing calcaneal osteotomy and TN arthrodesis versus revision of the malpositioned STJ fusion. Given the apex of deformity at the STJ arthrodesis site, the decision was made to take down the fusion and revise it. Wires were inserted along the STJ axis and a large saw was used to recreate the joint. The hindfoot was then pronated around the joint axis to reduce the iatrogenic varus deformity and fixed with a large-diameter screw.

Case 2. This patient had prior triple arthrodesis for the management of a talocalcaneal coalition as an adult **Fig. 7**. The patient was fused in a varus alignment and had symptoms of lateral ankle pain and lateral column overload with callus formation subfifth metatarsal.

Although the lateral talo-first metatarsal angle appears normal, the first ray clearly appears elevated in the frontal plane. Clinical examination confirmed this on a weight-bearing examination. This case exemplifies how one-dimensional radiographic measurements cannot necessarily account for torsional abnormalities.

CT scan images with three-dimensional rendering can provide insight on osseous relationship between hindfoot and forefoot, and assist with surgical planning. In this case, CT scanning provided further clarification of clinical suspicion.

Intraoperative flouroscan shows a lateralizing calcaneal osteotomy to correct the subtle hindfoot varus.

Guidewires are inserted along the previous TN and CC joint to plan for the derotational osteotomy. The previous hardware is left in temporarily to help guide the placement of the pins as the preoperative plain radiographs show that the TN joint was roughly at the center of the plate.

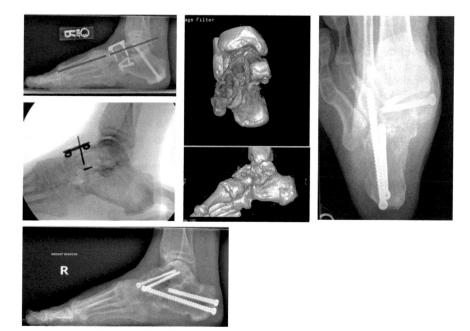

Fig. 7.

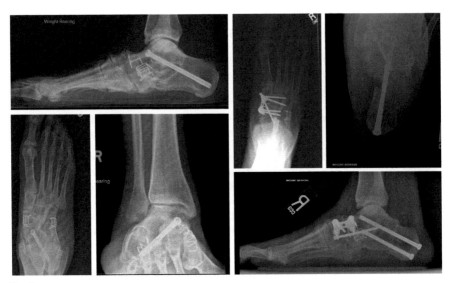

Fig. 8.

Postoperative radiographs show improved alignment in both planes. Note the placement of the hardware to maintain correction, specifically the utilization of a screw across the calcaneal osteotomy and lateral portion of the midtarsal osteotomy.

Case 3. This middle-aged man presented with painful, rigid flatfoot deformity **Fig. 8.** Patient states he had surgery during his childhood, although does not recall the indication or procedure. Based on history, a triple arthrodesis was most likely performed for a tarsal coalition.

Preoperative radiographs show progressive deformity through the NC joint with associated degenerative changes. Images of the ankle were obtained to confirm a congruent joint.

The patient underwent a medializing calcaneal osteotomy and corrective NC arthrodesis to address the multiplanar deformity. Patient also underwent a repeat gastrocnemius lengthening.

The osteotomy through the NC joint was carried to the lateral foot with a medial-based wedge to correct the abduction of the forefoot as well as plantarflex the medial column.

The calcaneal tuber was translated aggressively to restore the hindfoot under the tibial axis. Also note distal translation of the tuber to restore the calcaneal pitch.

SUMMARY

Inappropriate alignment of the foot after reconstructive flatfoot surgery can result in poor outcomes with recalcitrant pain. Identifying whether the foot has been under or over-corrected is paramount in addressing the pathology. Although there are no defined parameters to perform revision surgery, restoring alignment of the calcaneus under the long axis of the tibia and achieving a plantigrade foot will provide optimal outcomes. A thorough evaluation of underlying osseous deformity and muscle imbalances is vital in addressing all components of the deformity.

CLINICS CARE POINTS

- Identify whether the deformity is under- or overcorrected
  - Symptoms along the lateral column will typically represent overcorrection
  - Persistent symptoms along the medial foot and ankle represent undercorrection
- Appropriate imaging should include:
  - Weightbearing anteroposterior, medial oblique (AP, MO), and lateral foot x-rays
  - Ankle x-rays to assure the joint is congruent
  - Hindfoot alignment view
  - Advanced imaging can be beneficial in more complicated deformities
- Perform a thorough muscle inventory to address any dynamic deforming forces including equinus
- Correction should be performed through the apex of the deformity
  - This may require osteotomies or arthrodesis in multiple planes
- Restoration of the talo-first metatarsal angle both in the AP and lateral projection, and alignment of the calcaneus under the long axis of the tibia correlate with the ideal alignment of the foot

DISCLOSURE

The authors have no disclosures regarding conflicts of interest or commercial relationship in relation to the content of the work presented.

REFERENCES

1. Ford S, Scannell B. Pediatric flatfoot. Foot Ankle Clin 2017;22(3):643–56.
2. Dare D, Dodwell E. Pediatric flatfoot. Curr Opin Pediatr 2014;26(1):93–100.
3. Vulcano E, Maccario C, Myerson M. How to approach the pediatric flatfoot. World J Orthopedics 2016;7(1):1.
4. Day J, Kim J, Conti M, et al. Outcomes of idiopathic flexible flatfoot deformity reconstruction in the young patient. Foot Ankle Orthopaedics 2020;5(3). 247301142093798.
5. Johnson K, Strom D. Tibialis posterior tendon dysfunction. Clin Orthopaedics Relat Res 1989;239:196–206.
6. Abousayed M, Alley M, Shakked R, et al. Adult-acquired flatfoot deformity. JBJS Rev 2017;5(8):e7.
7. Henry J, Shakked R, Ellis S. Adult-acquired flatfoot deformity. Foot Ankle Orthopaedics 2019;4(1). 247301141882084.
8. Richie D. Biomechanics and orthotic treatment of the adult acquired flatfoot. Clin Podiatr Med Surg 2020;37(1):71–89.
9. Erard M, Sheean M, Sangeorzan B. Triple arthrodesis for adult-acquired flatfoot deformity. Foot Ankle Orthopaedics 2019;4(3). 247301141984960.
10. Conti M, Ellis S, Chan J, et al. Optimal position of the heel following reconstruction of the stage ii adult-acquired flatfoot deformity. Foot Ankle Int 2015;36(8):919–27.
11. Beischer A, Brodsky J, Polio F, et al. Functional outcome and gait analysis after triple or double arthrodesis. Foot Ankle Int 1999;20(9):545–53.
12. Röhm J, Zwicky L, Horn Lang T, et al. Mid- to long-term outcome of 96 corrective hindfoot fusions in 84 patients with rigid flatfoot deformity. Bone Joint J 2015; 97-B(5):668–74.

13. Irwin T. Overcorrected flatfoot reconstruction. Foot Ankle Clin 2017;22(3): 597–611.
14. Hunt K, Farmer R. The undercorrected flatfoot reconstruction. Foot Ankle Clin 2017;22(3):613–24.
15. Maenpaa H, Lehto M, Belt E. What went wrong in triple arthrodesis? Clin Orthopeadics Relate Res 2001;391:218–23.
16. Haddad SL, Myerson MS, Pell RF, et al. Clinical and radiographic outcome of revision surgery for failed triple arthrodesis. Foot Ankle Int 1997;18(8):489–99.
17. Toolan BC. Revision of failed triple arthrodesis with an opening-closing wedge osteotomy of the midfoot. Foot Ankle Int 2004;25(7):456–61.
18. de Cesar Netto C, Kunas GC, Soukup D. Correlation of clinical evaluation and radiographic hindfoot alignment in stage II adult-acquired flatfoot deformity. Foot Ankle Int 2018;39(7):771–9. SAGE Publications.
19. Cody EA, Williamson ER, Burket JC. Correlation of talar anatomy and subtalar joint alignment on weightbearing computed tomography with radiographic flatfoot parameters. Foot Ankle Int 2016;37(8):874–81. SAGE Publications.
20. Heckmann ND, Mercer JN, Wang LC, et al. Biomechanical evaluation of a cadaveric flatfoot model and lateral column lengthening technique. J Foot Ankle Surg 2021;60(5):956–9. Elsevier BV.
21. Meyr AJ, Matthew RW. Descriptive quantitative analysis of rearfoot alignment radiographic parameters. J Foot Ankle Surg 2015;54(5):860–71. Elsevier BV.
22. Rodriguez RP. Medial displacement calcaneal tuberosity osteotomy in the treatment of posterior tibial insufficiency. Foot Ankle Clin 2001;6(3):545–67. Elsevier BV.
23. Parupia Y, Klaver S, Merchant M. Pre and postoperative analysis of flatfoot reconstruction sparing the talonavicular joint. J Foot And Ankle Surg 2021;60(4):650–4. Elsevier BV.
24. Aiyer A, Dall G, Shub J, et al. Radiographic correction following reconstruction of adult acquired flatfoot deformity using the cotton medial cuneiform osteotomy. Foot Ankle Int 2016;37(5):508–13.

An Update on Pediatric Flatfoot

Caitlin Mahan Madden, DPM[a],*, Kieran T. Mahan, DPM, FCPP[b]

KEYWORDS

- Pes valgus • Calcaneal osteotomy • Metatarsus adductus • Arthroereisis
- Bone graft

KEY POINTS

- Planes of deformity must be evaluated before surgical planning.
- Surgical correction can be beneficial for the small group of patients with symptomatic flexible flatfoot that has failed conservative treatment.
- Multiple procedures exist for flatfoot correction and many can be combined for better correction.

INTRODUCTION

The pediatric pes valgus deformity is a distinct entity from the adult pes planus deformity, and must be evaluated and treated as such.

Using the terminology "pes valgus" helps to differentiate a pathologic, unstable low arch foot from a stable low arch foot that may be indicated by "pes planus" or "flatfoot." An asymptomatic stable but low arch foot does not need intervention. Indeed, children's feet typically do develop from flat to rectus,[1,2] and stability normally increases with age.[3] Patients who present with a symptomatic unstable deformity may require further evaluation and treatment.

EVALUATION

Although most adult pes planus patients present due to pain or disability, the pediatric patient is not always as straightforward. Younger children may be referred by a pediatrician or brought in by a parent concerned for "flat feet," or concerned that the patient "walks funny." Adolescents may complain of pain or difficulty with sports. Children may simply avoid sports or other vigorous activity. Patients may not be able to describe the duration or nature of their pain, as it has often been long-standing. The physical

[a] Private Practice, 708 West Nields Street, West Chester, PA 19382, USA; [b] Department of Surgery, Temple University School of Podiatric Medicine, 8th & Race Streets, Philadelphia, PA 19107, USA
* Corresponding author.
E-mail address: c.mahan.madden@gmail.com

Clin Podiatr Med Surg 40 (2023) 365–379
https://doi.org/10.1016/j.cpm.2022.11.006
0891-8422/23/© 2022 Elsevier Inc. All rights reserved.

examination must be in-depth to help provide information that may be missing from the standard patient interview.

A pathologic pes valgus deformity may result from several different causes. Equinus is certainly a common etiology, as a short tendo achillis, located on the pronating side of the subtalar joint, can be a powerful deforming force.[1] Compensating metatarsus adductus, internal tibial torsion, compensation for forefoot valgus or varus, and other deformities may be etiologies of rearfoot valgus. Ligamentous laxity, obesity, and other underlying medical conditions may also contribute to pes valgus.

Physical examination should include hip alignment and range of motion, knee alignment, tibial torsion, malleolar alignment, foot posture in stance and rest, gait evaluation, and range of motion of the ankle, rearfoot, and forefoot joints.[1] Heel raise will show an inversion of the heels and recreation of the medial arch in a flexible flatfoot. In a more rigid foot, inversion will not occur. Even in a flexible foot, if the deformity has been long-standing, inversion may not occur. Evaluation in stance may show significant transverse and frontal plane deformity (**Fig. 1**A, B). Gait examination may show a "too many toes sign" (which may sometimes be a presenting concern), adduction and plantarflexion of the talar head, early heel off, or other proximal angular or rotational deformities. A prominent navicular tuberosity or accessory navicular may be noted. Equinus should be evaluated. The Silfverskiold test can determine gastrocnemius equinus from gastrosoleal equinus. In addition, determining whether the deformity is rigid or flexible will guide further evaluation. A rigid deformity may be due to peroneal spasticity or a rearfoot or midfoot coalition. For peroneal spasticity, a common peroneal block or sinus tarsi block may assist in the evaluation. Radiographs are typically sufficient to visualize a coalition, although advanced imaging may be needed in cases where a fibrous coalition is suspected. Radiographs are not needed in all cases, but can be beneficial to evaluate the symptomatic pes valgus and are critical to the evaluation of the foot if surgery is being considered. These can help determine planes of deformity and compensation. The dorsal plantar radiograph will show degree of talar head uncovering, the talocalcaneal angle, and the cuboid abduction angle (**Fig. 2**). These indicate transverse plane compensation. This view also allows careful evaluation of the metatarsus adductus angle, which can be crucial when determining a surgical plan. Sagittal plane compensation can be seen on the lateral radiograph view, by examining the talar declination angle and the calcaneal inclination angle. Meary's angle (talo-first metatarsal angle) can also be measured on this view, and any navicular cuneiform fault can be observed. A calcaneal axial view can be used to evaluate the deformity of the calcaneus in the frontal plane and for a view of the middle and

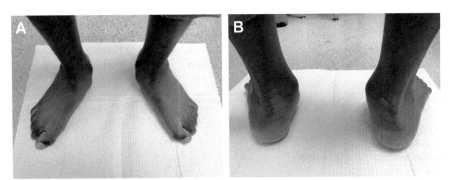

Fig. 1. (*A*) Stance evaluation showing transverse plane deformity with forefoot adduction. (*B*) Stance evaluation showing frontal plane deformity with rearfoot valgus.

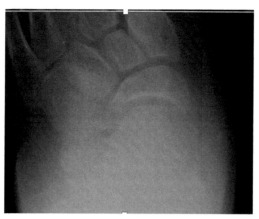

Fig. 2. Dorsoplantar radiograph showing a large degree of talar head uncovering.

posterior facets. A long leg axial view can be very helpful in evaluating the amount of rearfoot valgus. Computed tomography (CT) and MRI are not typically needed for the flexible pes valgus foot, although they may be useful for the rigid flatfoot or if there are other diagnostic concerns.

TREATMENT

The focus of this paper is on surgical treatment. However, it should be made very clear that most of the patients with a low arch do not require treatment and only a small minority of children with low arches require surgical treatment. The appearance of a flat foot does not necessitate treatment. "First do not harm" is the initial perspective that the clinician maintains when dealing with these patients. A symptomatic unstable foot may benefit from conservative care. A moderate to severe unstable foot, even when asymptomatic, may benefit from conservative care. Of those patients, a small number of patients who fail conservative care and/or those with a congenitally short tendo achillis may benefit from surgical correction. Some of those patients might be viewed as falling outside two standard deviations from the norm. There are quantitative data used by gait analysis laboratories such as the Malleolar Valgus Index (MVI) and/or the Center of Pressure Excursion Index (CPEI). The MVI measures static stance stability, whereas the CPEI measures dynamic stability.[4] These measurements are not commonly available in the practitioner's office. Clinical judgment becomes paramount along with radiographic documentation.

When considering surgical correction of the pes valgus foot, the planes of deformity must be carefully considered. "Planal Dominance" as illustrated by Green and Carol[5] is a theoretic way of looking at patients who may have different subtalar axes from the norm or "average". A transverse plane dominant foot, for example, has a vertical subtalar axis and compensates in the perpendicular plane, in this case, the transverse plane. These feet will have a high cuboid abduction angle, significant talar head uncovering, and a widened talocalcaneal angle. Similarly, saggital compensation occurs with a foot that has a more transverse axis. These feet may have a low calcaneal inclination angle, a plantarflexed talus, and a navicular cuneiform sag or elevated first metatarsal and/or unstable medial column joints. Again, a frontal plane foot has a longitudinal axis in the foot. This foot compensates with inversion and eversion. Although the "Planal Dominance" theory is an excellent way of helping to explain why we see some feet with deformity in one particular plane, things are not really that clear-cut. It is likely that just as there are few people with the so-called average subtalar joint axis of 42° elevated and 16° medial, so also it is unlikely that there are many, if any, patients who have subtalar axes with a purely vertical, horizontal or longitudinal axis. Consequently, deformities tend to be complex and multiplanar. The severity of the deformity may be compounded in multiplanar situations.

Despite all of the above, there are patients who would benefit from surgical treatment. Different surgical techniques can provide varying amounts of correction in each or multiple planes. The Cotton osteotomy increases arch height in the sagittal plane by providing first-ray plantarflexion. The Evans osteotomy provides powerful correction, largely in the transverse plane, although it is important to recognize that it is triplanar in correction. The Koutsogiannis, or medial calcaneal slide osteotomy, corrects frontal plane deformity. Achilles tendon or gastrocnemius lengthening procedures are used if there is underlying equinus. Typically, procedures are used in combination based on the amount of correction needed and the areas of deformity.

Evans Osteotomy

The Evans osteotomy provides correction of pes valgus by lengthening the lateral column.[6] This is largely corrective in the transverse plane, although sagittal and frontal plane correction also occurs.[7] The lengthening decreases subtalar joint protonation and also provides a slight decrease in overall subtalar joint motion, allowing for frontal plane correction. Lengthening the lateral column also creates increased tension along the long and short plantar ligaments, which provides sagittal plane correction due to plantarflexion of the forefoot on the rearfoot.[7] This can be seen in the increased calcaneal inclination angle on the lateral radiograph.[7] The transverse plane correction is seen clearly on an anterior-posterior radiograph with the realignment of the talonavicular joint, correction in the calcaneocuboid joint, and improvement in the talocalcaneal angle and the talo-first metatarsal angle.[7,8] Radiographic correction has been found to be predictable.[9,10]

Preoperative evaluation is important to identify the main planes of deformity and any other deformities. As noted, the Evans osteotomy is well-suited for correction of transverse plane deformity, such as those patients with a high subtalar axis and transverse plan compensation. These patients often fail orthotics and this deformity is not corrected well with medial column procedures alone. It is also crucial to determine if any metatarsus adductus is present. Lengthening the lateral column will exaggerate any underlying metatarsus adductus which can lead to complications or need for additional corrective procedures. This is particularly important for compensated metatarsus adductus, which may not be so apparent on first viewing. The best way to evaluate metatarsus adductus is with a neutral position radiograph. With the subtalar joint held in neutral position during the anteroposterior (AP) x-ray, any excessive metatarsus adductus is visible on the AP view. Failure to be aware of this can result in an excessively adducted foot. The Evans osteotomy can also make underlying equinus more evident, and posterior lengthening procedures are often needed to address this. Medial column procedures are also often needed to address sagittal or frontal plane deformities that are not fully corrected with the Evans.[9]

The Evans is an osteotomy of the anterior beak of the calcaneus, typically performed through an oblique or longitudinal incision. An oblique incision within the relaxed skin tension lines results in a finer scar. A longitudinal incision is less likely to disrupt the sural and intermediate dorsal cutaneous nerves as it parallels these. Whichever incision is chosen critical anatomy includes the relaxed skin tension lines, the peroneal tendons, the bifurcate ligament, the sural nerve, the intermediate dorsal cutaneous nerve, and the subtalar facets. For surgical technique, the extensor digitorum brevis is exposed and retracted dorsally, whereas the peroneal tendons and sural nerve are retracted inferiorly (**Fig. 3**). The calcaneocuboid joint is identified to help position the osteotomy; however, it is not opened and the bifurcate ligament is not sacrificed dorsally, which helps to preserve the stability of this joint. Ideally, the osteotomy is performed between the anterior and middle facets of the subtalar joint (**Fig. 4**A, B). This is typically 10 to 15 mm proximal to the calcaneocuboid joint. Anatomic variables in the subtalar joint can lead to damage to the middle facet and these must be carefully considered. In some cases the anterior and middle facets are contiguous.[11] An intraoperative C-arm view can be taken, using an instrument such as a freer elevator to mark the site of the planned osteotomy and ensure it will not violate the facets. Some have recommended a plantarflexion AP view of the foot to better visualize the anterior facet and the middle facet and sustentaculum tali. A guide wire can be used as a landmark for correct orientation of the osteotomy.[12] The osteotomy is made parallel to the calcaneocuboid joint and perpendicular to the weightbearing surface. In a cadaveric study evaluating the risk to the anterior and middle facets and the sustentaculum tali, Bussewitz and colleagues[13] recommended angling the osteotomy from posterolateral to anteromedial. This can be done either as a through-and-through cut, or as a modified wedge cut that preserves the medial hinge of the calcaneus. The complete osteotomy allows more correction while maintaining a medial hinge decreases the risk of displacement of the anterior beak and also decreases the risk of overcorrection. This also allows for better stability of the graft and thus more rapid healing. Once a graft has been chosen, a distractor or smooth lamina spreader can be placed to open the osteotomy and allow for graft placement. A bone tamp should be used to align the graft in its final position, to allow for more even distribution of forces and to decrease the risk of cracking the graft wall. It should be left slightly proud so it does not collapse within the cancellous bone of the calcaneus.

The Evans osteotomy was originally described with an autogenous tibial bone graft. Autograft is now often taken from the iliac crest rather than the tibia. The main benefits of autograft are the osteoinductive and osteoconductive properties; however, it comes with significant risks of donor site morbidity and pain. Allogeneic bone graft has also been shown to work well in this calcaneal osteotomy.[9,14] Allograft eliminates the risk of donor site complications and can also decrease surgical time with the advent of commercially available pre-fabricated and pre-sized grafts. The late Master clinician James Ganley DPM used tibial cortical pieces when he introduced the Evans procedure to the profession. At the Podiatry Institute in Tucker, Georgia, E. Dalton

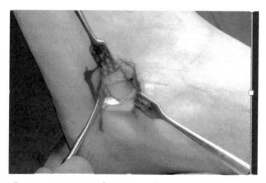

Fig. 3. Exposure for Evans osteotomy showing calcaneus with peroneal tendons and sural nerve retracted inferiorly.

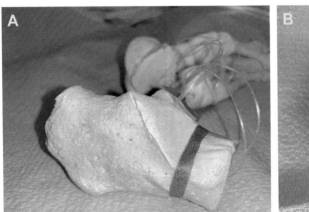
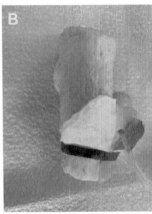

Fig. 4. (*A*) Lateral view of the calcaneus showing the posterior subtalar joint facet in yellow and the anterior and middle facets in orange and red, respectively. The location of the Evans osteotomy is shown in green. (*B*) Dorsal view of the calcaneus showing the location of the Evans osteotomy in green, between the anterior facet (*orange*) and the middle facet (*red*) of the subtalar joint.

McGlamry, another Master clinician, used allogeneic bone bank graft for the procedure. In a study of 300 bone grafts by Mahan and Hillstrom, some 146 were Evans osteotomy grafts where of those, only one was a delayed union, an extraordinary union rate.[14] The vascularity of the host site calcaneal bone is most likely the primary factor contributing to the high union rate. Prissel and Roukis conducted a review of studies that examined the incidence of nonunion of the unfixated, isolated Evans calcaneal osteotomy and showed how well bone grafts heal for this indication.[15] Autogenous bone can certainly be used and of course is superior to allogeneic bone. However, because of the rich vascular host site of the calcaneus, allogeneic bone can be used without adding the possible risks and time necessary to procure bone from the iliac crest, tibia, or calcaneus. Certainly, both materials are acceptable. Most often, when allogeneic bone is used for the graft it is a composite of cortical and cancellous bone, such as allogeneic tri-cortical iliac crest. This bone is strong enough to maintain the opening because of its tricortical nature, whereas the cancellous portion of the graft allows for rapid vascular ingrowth.

A surgeon can shape a tri-cortical wedge from allogeneic iliac crest, or use a pre-cut wedge of allogeneic bone. These typically come with an instrument set of sizers and tamps. These wedges are bi-cortical and may lack the strength of a tri-cortical wedge. Although there is some theoretic concern for increased nonunion rate with an allograft, research has not shown a significant difference in nonunion rates for the Evans osteotomy.[15]

Graft shape and size is also a major consideration. Grafts can be rectangular, triangular, or truncated wedges. Different shapes and sizes can affect both the amount of correction and the risk of certain complications. In a finite-element modeling study by Wu and colleagues,[16] rectangular grafts showed better tarsal realignment; however, they caused increased pressure at the calcaneocuboid joint and increased strain along the spring ligament with increasing size. They also changed the contact areas across the calcaneocuboid joint and talonavicular joint. Triangular wedges showed decreased changes in the biomechanical forces across the calcaneocuboid and talonavicular joints when compared with rectangular wedges of the same sizes, along with better maintenance of contact areas. Care must be taken when choosing a graft size as well. Too large a graft can lead to overcorrection, causing increased plantarflexion of the forefoot on the rearfoot and increased pressure at the calcaneocuboid joint, and can increase the risk of anterior beak shift due to increased tension on the long and short plantar ligaments. Too small a graft can lead to undercorrection with continued deformity despite adjunct procedures. However, it must be remembered that less than full correction radiographically is not the same as clinical undercorrection. The goal of the procedure should be to create a controllable foot, rather than a "normal" foot on radiograph. Evaluating the realignment of the talonavicular joint is the best basis for determining the amount of correction needed for a patient. Typically the authors use grafts that are 8 to 9 mm truncated wedges, although this may vary based on the individual. Experience has shown that slightly smaller grafts, or decreased correction due to graft resorption, have not led to significant negative clinical results, whereas larger graft sizes are more likely to lead to issues due to overcorrection.

In more recent years, various companies have developed titanium wedges and wedge-locking plates to be used in place of bone grafts. In addition, some surgeons who still use bone graft now fixate the graft to keep it in place, although traditionally the graft was press-fit and did not use fixation.[17] The expansion of methods has led to more research regarding the potential benefits and complications regarding these.

Porous titanium wedges are felt to have several benefits over autograft or allograft. They are inert and do not carry the risk of donor-associated infection. The physical properties are similar to subchondral bone. The titanium is stronger than bone and cannot be resorbed. In a study by Matthews and colleagues,[18] porous titanium wedges showed no significant changes in radiographic measurements after correction over a long-term follow-up. Furthermore, 100% of grafts incorporated and none required removal. Therefore, porous titanium wedges are a reasonable alternative to autograft or allograft. However, they are certainly subject to complications including need for graft removal (**Fig. 5**A, B).

Wedge-locking plates are another alternative to bone graft. Similar to titanium wedges, one of the goals of these plates is to better maintain mid-calcaneal length long term. A study by Protzman and colleagues[19] showed less decrease in mid-calcaneal length in a group of patients with wedge locking plates compared with tricortical wedge allograft at 6 months, although results at 3 months were similar between the two groups. Patients in both groups developed displacement of the anterior calcaneal process, although at different points. The allograft wedge group showed displacement at 3-month follow-up, whereas the wedge locking plate group showed displacement at an immediate postoperative radiograph. Although fixation is often used to help prevent anterior calcaneal process displacement, care must be taken to ensure proper alignment intraoperatively.

DeHeer and colleagues[17] reviewed results after locking plate fixation across the graft. Locking plates are felt to provide better angular stability, to prevent anterior displacement of the anterior calcaneal process. They are also felt to maintain the length of the lateral column as the graft incorporates. Their study noted a 30% hardware removal rate in a total of 70 feet, with more females than males developing painful hardware. Age and laterality did not affect the rate of hardware removal. Mosca in 1995 recommended pinning across the calcaneocuboid joint, anterior calcaneal fragment, and graft, to decrease the risk of displacement of the anterior beak and increase the stability of the graft.[20] Attia and colleagues[21] showed that Steinmann pin fixation across the calcaneocuboid joint led to an increased risk of arthritic changes in this joint when the pin was left in place and removed postoperatively, as opposed to being removed during surgery.

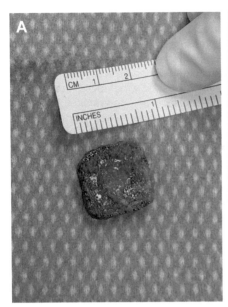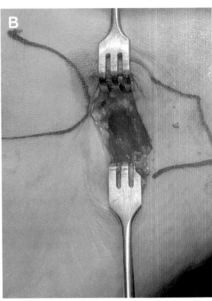

Fig. 5. (*A*) Titanium wedge Evans graft explanted due to pain and dorsal displacement. (*B*) Site of previous titanium wedge graft, now prepared for placement of cadaveric bone graft.

Complications of the Evans osteotomy include nonunion of the graft site, displacement of the anterior calcaneal tuberosity, invasion of the subtalar joint, sural nerve and/or peroneal tendon injury, under- or overcorrection, and increased calcaneocuboid pressures which can lead to lateral foot pain, stress fractures of the fifth metatarsal, and calcaneocuboid joint arthritis. Nonunion is uncommon, with frequency ranging around 4% to 5%, although some studies have shown it to be even lower.[15,22] The rich vascularization of the calcaneus is felt to be a large factor in the very low rate of nonunion. In addition, the changes in the mechanic forces after correction, including the restoration of the windlass mechanism of the plantar fascia, help to maintain a press-fit graft in place, decreasing the risk of motion and nonunion.[23] Dorsal displacement of the anterior calcaneal tuberosity is a more frequent complication (**Fig. 6**). The tightening of lateral soft tissues is felt to put additional stress on the anterior calcaneus, squeezing it dorsally. Dunn and Meyer retrospectively reviewed unfixated osteotomies and found that significant dorsal displacement at 6 weeks went on to resolve upon longer follow-up. Improvements in talar declination angle and calcaneal inclination angle were seen at first postoperative follow-up and continued into the late postoperative period.[24] Multiple studies have proposed fixating the anterior calcaneal process, typically with Kirshner wires or Steinmann pins across the calcaneocuboid joint.[12,20,21] Fixation does not seem to significantly reduce the rate or magnitude of displacement.[25] The union rate is already quite high with these osteotomies, so the principal benefit to fixation with a plate seems to be less graft resorption. To what degree that is clinically significant is not clear. Increased pressure along the lateral column after calcaneal lengthening can lead to stress fractures of the fifth metatarsal and lateral column pain. Ellis and colleagues[26] reported an 11.2% incidence of plantar lateral pain in 132 feet after Evans osteotomy. In a separate smaller study, patients were found to have increased plantar pressures specifically in the lateral midfoot, which may account for lateral column pain after lateral column lengthening.[27] As a

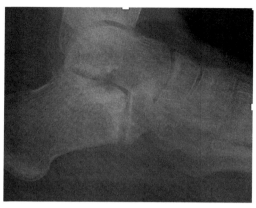

Fig. 6. Lateral radiograph showing dorsal displacement of the anterior calcaneal process following Evans osteotomy.

larger graft will increase lateral column pressures more, using a smaller graft size is felt to reduce the risk of lateral column pain postoperatively. For patients with more severe deformity, multiple procedures should be used for correction rather than relying solely on the Evans. Graft shape and size both influence the degree of correction. A wedged piece will result in the least correction, with a truncated wedge resulting in greater correction and a rectangular piece resulting in the greatest correction. For each of those shapes, correction will vary depending upon the lateral width of the graft. For example, a 10-mm graft will produce greater correction than a 7-mm graft. Balancing the size and shape of the graft to get the ideal correction is a matter of both art and science. Excessive correction can lead to subtalar joint jamming, an inverted heel, insufficient pronatory motion in the subtalar joint, and subtalar and lateral pain. Because this is usually an elective procedure, it is important to err on the side of under-correction, a lesson that has been learned since this procedure was first used in the late 1970s. In addition to graft size and shape, the osteotomy can be performed as a through-and-through osteotomy, as is typically done, or can be performed as an opening wedge osteotomy with the medial hinge intact. A wedge osteotomy, as opposed to the typical distraction lengthening, will usually create less overall correction. On the contrary, there is less risk of overcorrection with this technique and the anterior beak is more stable. In situations where there is less deformity, a wedge osteotomy with the medial hinge intact is a viable option.

Cotton Osteotomy

The Cotton osteotomy is an opening wedge osteotomy of the medial cuneiform that provides plantarflexion of the first ray. It does not address hypermobility at the navicular cuneiform joint or first metatarsal cuneiform joint, but it does address the structural elevation of the first ray. It is technically on the simpler side and relatively quick to perform and is thus a popular adjunct procedure in flatfoot correction.

The longitudinal incision is centered over the medial cuneiform, parallel to the extensor hallucis longus (EHL) tendon. It is carried through the superficial fascia, using careful dissection to avoid destabilizing the proximal and distal joints of the medial cuneiform. Intraoperative x-ray can be helpful with this and with incision placement. Once the position is confirmed, a periosteal incision is made transversely in the same direction as the osteotomy. It is placed in the area of the distal two-thirds of the cuneiform. The osteotomy is performed with a sagittal saw, with care taken to retract and protect the EHL from the saw. An osteotome is then used to wedge open the cut, with the goal of keeping the plantar hinge intact. The plantar cortex must be sufficiently thinned before use of the osteotome, otherwise, the force can cause an intra-articular fracture into the first metatarsal cuneiform joint. Similar to an Evans osteotomy, sets are available with sizers and pre-shaped grafts, which can be used to determine and place the appropriate graft. Typically graft sizes range from 4 to 6 mm, although this varies with the degree of deformity and the size of an individual's foot. When determining graft size, care must be taken to not cause excessive plantarflexion, as this can lead to painful sesamoiditis. Fixation is not typically necessary, although some surgeons use small plates. Titanium wedges and wedge locking plates are also available for the Cotton osteotomy, as they are for the Evans. Cook and colleagues[18] evaluated the safety and efficacy of 63 porous titanium wedges in both Evans and Cotton osteotomies, and found them to provide durable correction with a low risk of complications. Fraser and colleagues[28] found similar short-term results in a study focusing on titanium wedges in Cotton osteotomies without Evans osteotomies, although their cases did include other adjunct procedures.

Because the Cotton is typically used as an adjunctive procedure, it can be difficult to fully assess its effect on alignment. Studies have typically used Meary's angle (lateral talo-first metatarsal angle) as an indicator of the correction obtained after a Cotton osteotomy.[29–31] Complications following this procedure include nonunion, delayed union, graft displacement, neuritis, and need for revision surgery or hardware removal. Nonunion and delayed union are generally felt to be rare.[30] Graft displacement even without fixation is also felt to be uncommon. Au and colleagues[31] examined maintenance of correction in short- and long-term postoperative follow-up. They found a loss of radiographic correction at the 6- to 10-week and 10- to 16-week follow-up periods, which corresponded to the start of weightbearing at 6 weeks. There was not any indication of clinical manifestations due to loss of correction. They hypothesized that further study of porous titanium wedges would show the better-maintained correction. Neuritis can be seen due to injury to the medial dorsal cutaneous nerve. The medial dorsal cutaneous nerve runs obliquely across the medial cuneiform, from proximal lateral to distal medial. Thus the standard Cotton incision, placed longitudinally over the medial cuneiform, puts this nerve at risk. It is often encountered during dissection and must be retracted for protection during the osteotomy and graft placement, and fixation if used. Boffeli and Schnell reported a modified incision, running obliquely over the medial cuneiform medial and parallel to the palpable medial dorsal cutaneous nerve. This allows the nerve to remain protected within the dorsal lateral soft tissues.[32] However, the success of this incision placement relies on accurate palpation of the medial dorsal cutaneous nerve.

Medial Calcaneal Slide/Koutsogiannis

The medial calcaneal slide osteotomy is a through-and-through osteotomy through the posterior calcaneus from the lateral side. Its correction arises from the shift of the tendo achillis from the pronating side of the subtalar axis to the supinating side of the axis. This decreases the valgus deformity of the calcaneus by helping to make the inverting muscles have a greater mechanical advantage and helps to support the medial longitudinal arch.[33] It works well for the compensated metatarsus adductus foot type, where an Evans osteotomy might adduct the foot too much. It is also frequently used in combination with the Evans (**Fig. 7**).[1]

The procedure starts with a curvilinear incision laterally, posterior to the peroneal tendons (**Fig. 8**A). Care must be taken to avoid the sural nerve in this area. The periosteum is then incised. Fixation can be accomplished with posterior to anterior screws

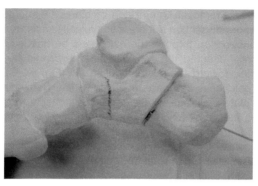

Fig. 7. Bone model showing placement of Evans osteotomy and completed medial calcaneal slide osteotomy.

or with lateral step-off plates. If screws are used, the periosteal dissection is minimal, although these cannot be used in patients with open growth plates. For lateral plating systems, more periosteal dissection is performed with a key elevator (**Fig. 8**B). The peroneal tendons should be retracted anteriorly for plates. Intraoperative x-ray can confirm the location and direction of the osteotomy, ensuring the cut is not too proximal or too distal, which could risk invasion of the posterior facet of the subtalar joint. Crego elevators can be used at the superior and inferior sides of the osteotomy. Once the bone cut has been made with power instrumentation and checked with an osteotome, the Crego elevators can be removed which allows the osteotomy to shift (**Fig. 8**C). The shift is typically 6 to 10 mm and is fixated with a temporary pin (**Fig. 8**D, E). The position is checked under intraoperative x-ray. Fixation is then accomplished as noted. For posterior screws, one or two (vertically stacked) screws can be used, typically larger (6.5 mm) headless cannulated screws, with careful attention to countersinking to help reduce the need for hardware removal. Headed screws

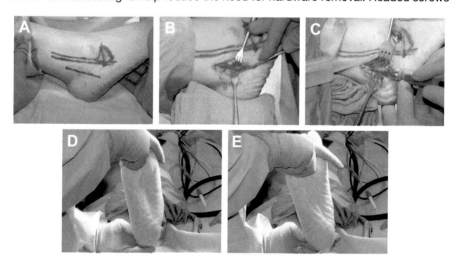

Fig. 8. (*A*) Incision placement for medial calcaneal slide osteotomy. Note outline of peroneal tendon course, anterior calcaneus, and incision for Evans osteotomy. (*B*) Key elevator used to shift periosteum before bone cut. (*C*) The osteotomy is made perpendicular to the bone and parallel to the posterior facet. (*D*) Position before osteotomy shift. (*E*) Position after osteotomy shift.

are more likely to require removal. Lateral step-off plates are another good fixation option. They require more dissection but are also typically easier to locate and remove should future reconstruction through the calcaneus be needed. One such system uses a locking screw directed through the plate perpendicular to the calcaneus, with another directed toward the sustentaculum tali (**Fig. 9**A–C). If prominent, the lateral side of the calcaneus can be tamped down flat. Care must be taken during closure to ensure plate coverage with the superficial fascia to promote good scar mobility. Protecting the tarsal tunnel during the procedure is important. There is a version of this procedure that uses a minimal incision approach.

The "double calcaneal osteotomy" involves a Koutsogiannis and an Evans, performed together. This has proven useful for both adolescent pes valgus patients and adult patients with reducible deformities.[33]

Arthroereisis

Arthroereisis is an option that is well-suited for the truly flexible pes valgus deformity. Excessive eversion is limited by placing an implant within the sinus tarsi, which blocks abnormal motion of the talus while still allowing inversion.[34] The benefits of this procedure include it being less invasive, and having a short healing time and a low complication rate. Specific risks with arthroereisis include sinus tarsi pain, implant extrusion, and a possible need for device removal or exchange. Over- or undercorrection is also possible.[35] It is typically used in pre-adolescent patients, as many younger children experience spontaneous resolution of symptomatic pes valgus, and older patients may not have sufficient time for the remodeling of hindfoot bones and ligaments that allows for more durable correction.[36]

Surgically, the procedure starts by identifying the sinus tarsi from the lateral aspect with a 27-gauge needle, approximately 1 cm anterior and inferior from the tip of the lateral malleolus. Once the sinus tarsi is identified, a small 1.5 cm incision is made overlying it, following the relaxed skin tension lines. This should allow for avoidance of the sural nerve and the intermediate dorsal cutaneous nerve. Blunt dissection is performed through the subcutaneous tissue and deep fascia with a mosquito hemostat. The cannula rod from the arthroereisis set is then placed into and across the sinus tarsi. Tenting of the medial skin will indicate that the rod has passed the whole distance. Some sets have a dilation device that can then be placed over the cannula rod and inserted with a gentle twisting motion, to allow for stretching of the sinus tarsi. The implant sizers are then trialed. With each sizer subtalar eversion should be evaluated and intraoperative dorsoplantar and lateral radiographs taken. The correct sizer

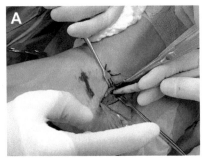
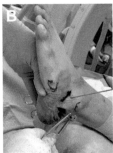
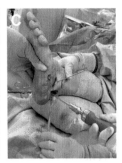

Fig. 9. (*A*) Lateral calcaneus prepared for osteotomy and plate application. Note the amount of periosteal dissection. (*B*) Placement of lateral step-off plate after temporary fixation with a *K*-wire. (*C*) Screws are inserted in the lateral step-off plate.

will limit eversion to 2° to 4°, and on radiograph the medial edge of the sizer will sit at the midline of the talus. Once the correct size is determined, the sizer is removed and the corresponding sized implant is placed over the cannula rod and inserted with a driver. Intraoperative radiographs are taken to ensure proper final positioning. After removal of the driver and rod the area is irrigated and closed.

Although arthroereisis can be a good surgical option, it does lack the corrective power of some of the other osseous procedures. A 2019 study conducted a systemic review to examine lateral column lengthening versus arthroereisis. They found that lateral column lengthening led to greater radiographic improvements and greater improvements in functional outcome scores. There were similar rates of re-operation and patient satisfaction. The arthroereisis group did show a lower rate of complications.[36] Each procedure has specific advantages. Lateral column lengthening allows for greater correction in feet with severe forefoot abduction, and can be used in a wider age range. Arthroereisis is typically used in children between 8 and 12 years of age with moderate forefoot abduction and particularly excessive subtalar eversion.

SUMMARY

Pes valgus deformity is frequently encountered in the pediatric population. There are several surgical approaches that are successful in correcting this. Multiple planes of deformity can exist and all must be properly addressed. Tendo achillis lengthening may be required. Stability must be achieved in the rearfoot and the medial column. The goal of surgical correction should focus on pain reduction and producing a controllable foot with a reduction of deforming forces. The need for some flexibility and adaptability of the foot must be balanced with the need for controlling excess protonation.

CLINICS CARE POINTS

- Surgical planning should address all planes of deformity.
- Check position for Evans osteotomy under C-arm to ensure avoidance of the anterior and middle facets.
- Use caution with larger Evans grafts.
- Do not overly plantarflex the first ray with a Cotton graft as this can lead to sesamoid pain.
- Choose incision placement carefully when performing both an Evans and a medial calcaneal slide.
- Do not use posterior to anterior screws for a medial calcaneal slide through an open growth plate.
- Consider arthroeresis for the very flexible foot in younger patients.

DISCLOSURE

Neither author has any commercial or financial conflicts of interest to disclose.

REFERENCES

1. Mahan KT, Madden CM. Pediatric and adolescent pes valgus deformity The pediatric foot and ankle. Switzerland: Springer Nature; 2020. p. 169–90.

2. Staheli LT. Evaluation of planovalgus foot deformities with special reference to the natural history. J Am Podiatr Med Assoc 1987;77(1):2–6.

3. Napolitano C, Walsh S, Mahoney L, et al. Risk factors that may adversely modify the natural history of the pediatric pronated foot. Clin Podiatr Med Surg 2000; 17(3):397–417.

4. Song J, Hillstrom HJ, Secord D. Levitt J foot type biomechanics: comparison of planus and rectus foot types. JAPMA 1996;86(1):16–23.

5. Green DR, Carol A. Planal dominance. JAPA 1984;74(2):98–103. PMID 6707427.

6. Evans D. Calcaneo-valgus deformity. J Bone Joint Surg Br 1975;57(3):270–8.

7. Lamm BM, Knight J, Ernst JJ. Evans calcaneal osteotomy: assessment of multi-plantar correction. JFAS 2021. https://doi.org/10.1053/j.jfas.2020.10.016.

8. Dollard MD, Marcinko DE, Lazerson A, et al. The Evans calcaneal osteotomy for correction of flexible flatfoot syndrome. J Foot Surg 1984;23(4):291–301.

9. Mahan KT, McGlamry ED. Evans calcaneal osteotomy for flexible pes valgus deformity. A preliminary study. Clin Podiatr Med Surg 1987;4(1):137–51. PMID 2949808.

10. Sangeorzan B, Mosca V, Hansen S. Effect of calcaneal lengthening on relation-ships among the hind foot, mid foot and forefoot. Foot & Ankle 1993;14(3): 136–41.

11. Mosca VS, Ragab AA, Stewart SL, et al. Implications of subtalar joint anatomic variation in calcaneal lengthening osteotomy. J Pediatr Orthop 2003;23:79–83.

12. Sapogovskiy A, Hassanein MY, Kenis V. Lateral column lengthening revisited: a simple intraoperative approach to ensure a true extra-articular osteotomy. JFAS 2020;59:1318–21.

13. Bussewitz BW, DeVries JG, Hyer CF. Evans osteotomy and risk to subtalar joint articular facets and sustentaculum tali: a cadaver study. JFAS 2013;52:594–7.

14. Mahan KT, Hillstrom HJ. Bone grafting in foot and ankle surgery. J Am Podiatr Med Assoc 1998;88(3):109–18.

15. Prissel M. Roukis TS Incidence of nonunion of the unfixed, isolated Evans calca-neal osteotomy: a systematic review. JFAS 2012;51:323–5.

16. Wu J, Liu H, Xu C. Biomechanical effects of graft shape for the Evans lateral col-umn lengthening procedure: a patient-specific finite element investigation. Foot Ankle Int 2022;43(3):404–13.

17. DeHeer PA, Patel S, Standish SN. Procedure specific hardware removal after Evans osteotomy. J Am Podiatr Med Assoc 2020;110(2):1–7.

18. Matthews M, Cook EA, Cook J, et al. Long-term outcomes of corrective osteoto-mies using porous titanium wedges for flexible flatfoot deformity correction. JFAS 2018;57:924–30.

19. Protzman NM, Wobst GM, Storts EC, et al. Mid-calcaneal length after Evans calcaneal osteotomy: a retrospective comparison of wedge locking plates and tri-cortical allograft wedges. JFAS 2015;54:900–4.

20. Mosca VS. Calcaneal lengthening for valgus deformity of the hindfoot. Results in children who had severe, symptomatic flatfoot and skewfoot. J Bone Jt Surg Am 1995;77(4):500–12.

21. Attia E, Heldt B, Roepe IG, et al. Does the stabilization of the calcaneocuboid joint with Steinmann pin in Evans osteotomy affect its incidence of arthritis? Foot 2021; 49:101846.

22. Jara ME. Evans osteotomy complications. Foot Ankle Clin N Am 2017;22:573–85.

23. Hicks JH. The Mechanics of the foot. II. The plantar aponeurosis and the arch. J Anat 1954;88(1):25–30.

24. Dunn SP, Meyer J. Displacement of the anterior process of the calcaneus after Evans calcaneal osteotomy. JFAS 2011;50(4):402–6.
25. Adams SB, Simpson AW, Pugh LI, et al. Calcaneocuboid joint subluxation after calcaneal lengthening for planovalgus foot deformity in children with cerebral palsy. J Pediatr Orthop 2009;29(2):170–4.
26. Ellis SJ, Williams BR, Garg R, et al. Incidence of plantar lateral foot pain before and after the use of trial metal wedges in lateral column lengthening. Foot Ankle Int 2011;32(7):665–73.
27. Ellis SJ, Yu JC, Johnson AH, et al. Plantar pressures in patients with and without lateral foot pain after lateral column lengthening. J Bone Joint Surg Am 2010; 92(1):81–91.
28. Fraser TW, Kadakia AR, Doty JF. Complications and early radiographic outcomes of flatfoot deformity correction with metallic midfoot opening wedge implants. Foot & Ankle Orthopaedics 2019;4(3):1–5.
29. Boffeli TJ, Schnell KR. Cotton osteotomy in flatfoot reconstruction: a review of consecutive cases. JFAS 2017;56:990–5.
30. Lutz M, Myerson M. Radiographic analysis of an opening wedge osteotomy of the medial cuneiform. Foot Ankle In 2011;32(3):278–87.
31. Au B, Patel NB, Smith CN, et al. Short- to intermediate-term radiographic outcomes following Cotton osteotomy. JFAS 2021;S1067-2516(21):00486–95. Online ahead of print.
32. Boffeli TJ, Schnell KR. Cotton osteotomy in flatfoot reconstruction: a case reports highlighting surgical technique and modified incision to protect the medial dorsal cutaneous nerve. JFAS 2017;56:874–84.
33. Catanzariti AR, Mendicino RW, King GL, et al. Double calcaneal osteotomy: realignment considerations in eight patients. J Am Pod Med Assoc 2005; 95(1):53–9.
34. Pavone V, Costarella L, Testa G, et al. Calcaneo-stop procedure in the treatment of the juvenile symptomatic flatfoot. J Foot Ankle Surg 2013;52(4):444–7.
35. Needleman RL. Current topic review: subtalar arthroereisis for the correction of flexible flatfoot. Foot Ankle Int 2005;26(4):336–46.
36. Suh DH, Park JH, Lee SH, et al. Lateral column lengthening versus subtalar arthroereisis for paediatric flatfeet: a systematic review. Int Orthop 2019. https://doi.org/10.1007/s00264-019-04303-3.

Moving?

Make sure your subscription moves with you!

To notify us of your new address, find your **Clinics Account Number** (located on your mailing label above your name), and contact customer service at:

Email: journalscustomerservice-usa@elsevier.com

800-654-2452 (subscribers in the U.S. & Canada)
314-447-8871 (subscribers outside of the U.S. & Canada)

Fax number: 314-447-8029

**Elsevier Health Sciences Division
Subscription Customer Service
3251 Riverport Lane
Maryland Heights, MO 63043**

*To ensure uninterrupted delivery of your subscription, please notify us at least 4 weeks in advance of move.

ELSEVIER